MW01175154

LAUNCHING
SOLO

◆ FriesenPress

Suite 300 - 990 Fort St
Victoria, BC, V8V 3K2
Canada

www.friesenpress.com

ISBN
978-1-5255-8572-2 (Hardcover)
978-1-5255-8571-5 (Paperback)
978-1-5255-8573-9 (eBook)

1. FAMILY & RELATIONSHIPS, AGING

Distributed to the trade by The Ingram Book Company

Bob Cowin

Launching Solo

The First Year of
Single People's Retirement

BOB COWIN

For Maureen

TABLE OF CONTENTS

CURIOSITY

The advertisements feature a distinguished couple—tall and trim, well-tailored, and sporting sizable swatches of grey at their temples—strolling hand in hand at water's edge along a tropical beach. Palm trees frame the sunny tableau, with calm, azure waters forming the backdrop. Their faces glow, giving no indication of boredom after weeks of idling in the sand and surf.

And then there are the retirement announcements that periodically grace office newsletters. "After a zillion years of wonderful service with Scrooge, Cratchit & Company, Kelly is moving on to concentrate on her golf game." At least, she'll frequent the greens during the six months each year when it's pleasant to linger outside. Perhaps three days a week if she's keen.

As charming as the dreams and mythologies of retirement may be, they don't necessarily reflect the reality of people who have recently launched into this next phase of life. We're well aware that the senior years are every bit as complex and variable as any other stage of life, but somehow our society is not very good at describing and anticipating all the emotions—the ups and downs, the surprises and the predictable—that come with stepping over the retirement threshold. A wide range of articles and seminars make a valiant effort to prepare us, but all too often, the transition proves bumpier than anticipated.

I developed an interest in the first year of retirement, and in the experiences of single people in particular, during my Saturday morning yoga class. It's a neighbourhood session, held in a church hall on a casual, drop-in basis. The instructor, Megan, is a nurse who enrolled in yoga teacher training as a mid-life hobby with the potential to develop into a sideline during her retirement. She also registered in a craft beer and brewing program through the continuing education department of our local university for much the same reason, but that's another story.

Health care is a challenging industry, and over a two-year period, I increasingly noticed Megan's weariness with her latest crop of managers. It's not that they were especially dysfunctional, but one's patience wears thin when one has been through several similar iterations in previous years. Megan knew it was time to get out before cynicism consumed her. It was just a question of determining exactly when to leave.

Megan did her retirement homework. She attended financial planning seminars. She maintained and nurtured a healthy social network. She had her hobbies. She recognized that retirement is a major transition and prepared for the foreseeable psychological challenges. As far as I could tell, she was doing everything right, and I sometimes mentioned this when we chatted about her work and post-employment plans.

Which we did regularly.

After the third consecutive Saturday of hearing exactly the same description of her retirement preparations, it finally dawned on me that Megan was far more anxious than she was letting on. I took this to be a healthy sign, evidence that she was being realistic and sensible, because Megan lives alone in a large city with few family members close by. When you're single in these circumstances, your job naturally becomes a significant part of your life and identity. Retirement becomes a really big deal. And so, I listened and encouraged her as best I could. She is, after all, an appealing person, the type for whom you wish the best.

Eventually, Megan selected a date, and the tenor of our conversations shifted. Still a textbook example of how to prepare, she arranged to become a very part-time research assistant for several months after retirement in a couple of projects that excited her. This would ensure some connection with a few valued colleagues, a way of making her departure from the workplace a little less abrupt.

The big day came and went, essentially as planned. The substitute yoga instructor during Megan's celebratory trip to Peru was agreeable, but we were all happy to welcome Megan back after her travels. Our conversations continued because I have tight body tissues and usually linger after class for extra stretching. I'm faithful about this because, although it's not exactly the fountain of youth, maintaining my flexibility seems to be a powerful anti-aging strategy for me.

Most Saturdays, we just nattered while Megan gathered her yoga props and I elongated. Often, the conversation concerned the activities of the past week or what was on the calendar for the coming days. One morning, the exchange took a different turn. "I'm thinking I'll maybe spend a bit of time in Victoria," said Megan.

"That's a lovely city," I replied. "I studied there for a couple of years and would have liked to stay longer. The only job I could find, though, was on the mainland, and I've been here ever since. But I still love it each time I take the ferry and disembark in Victoria."

"What about spending a few months there?" Megan probed. "Do you think you could move there permanently?"

"Yes, I'm sure I'd like it. Is that what you're talking about? Moving there and not just visiting?"

"Maybe. Perhaps do a trial run next autumn, and not simply uproot irrevocably from here. I could rent out my condo and use the money towards a temporary place on Vancouver Island to see how I like it."

Megan went on to explain how her life, while satisfying, was fragmented. "I have plenty of friends, but they often live thirty or sixty minutes away. They typically don't know each other. My biking buddies are not the same people I go to the theatre with. I'm hoping that if I were in a smaller city with a high percentage of active seniors like me, I might develop a more robust social network. Friends who could be something of a tribe. Friends who live close enough that we could do spur-of-the-moment things together. Maybe I'm a small-town girl at heart."

At least, that's how I recall our discussions. I eventually checked back with Megan to find out what she had really said. Her version appears in the next chapter. In the meantime, my understanding of her story got me thinking. Several people came to mind who had been so focused on leaving toxic jobs that they gave little thought to what their post-employment life might look like. They struggled during those first months of retirement, although they seem to be finding their rhythm now. But they were married and had supportive spouses. How, I wondered, would they have fared if they had been on their own like Megan?

Another person had remarked to me, "It was the second six months of retirement that I found hard. The beginning was fine." I hadn't pursued that comment, but neither did I forget it. Now, I wanted to follow-up and learn what had prompted it.

I poked around the Internet and rifled through library catalogues, but it wasn't as easy to find information about the experiences of single people in their first year of retirement as I had hoped. Such information does, of course, exist, but it didn't exactly whack me in the face. So, while continuing my research, I started casually asking people about their retirement experiences. They were eager to talk and had plenty of interest to share. Despite hearing stories that were highly individual and varied, a common thread of humanity wove them together in ways that resonated with me. And so, I started writing down their stories, the genesis of what eventually became this book.

I didn't want to produce a *how-to* book full of earnest advice or to analyze individuals' experiences to any great extent. Neither did I care how it was that someone happened to be single when they finished working. Whether the single state was due to never having married, divorce, or death didn't matter to me. Just that they were entering retirement all on their own.

My motivation was simply to gain a better sense of

what actually happens in the initial months of retirement, especially the extent to which circumstances vary from person to person. I hope you'll find the resulting stories and observations to be as fascinating as I did. I've changed names and taken liberties with the details and dialogue, but the following accounts faithfully relate the essence of what people told me. Although the resulting themes and issues may have come from a specific set of individuals, they strike me as food for thought for just about everybody launching into retirement.

MEGAN

I finally caught up with Megan, my middle-aged yoga instructor with a real person's body, to hear an extended version of her retirement story. She didn't say a thing this time about testing the waters in Victoria for a few months. I suppose that, like adolescence, this stage of life is a good one for exploring and tossing out ideas, making false starts, and eventually settling into a path that works. In any event, she did recap how her views about friendships have shifted now that she is no longer in the working world.

"Could you remind me what you were saying a few weeks ago about your friendships evolving?" I had prompted.

"Evolving?"

"Well, maybe that's not the right word. I think it's more along the lines that you're finding the people you'd like to spend time with are not quite the same as you expected."

Megan's blank look transformed. "Oh, I know what you're asking about. I've had people in my life who were really just acquaintances, people I'd see only once in a while. I was often the instigator, and that took energy. I'm dropping those who don't reciprocate, while reconnecting with folks whose circumstances may also have changed, making it easier for us to get together on weekdays."

She elaborated, "Some people I enjoy spending time with live far away. Even meeting midway for a meal can require a substantial drive. It takes planning, and the engagement turns into a half-day event. I hadn't thought about this before because we had previously connected at work. There, you're already together and can do things at lunch or after hours. Now, I'm trying to find more local connections, not that I'm going to drop everybody else."

She spoke more pensively now, idly fingering the mauve fabric of her sweater. "Some of those former acquaintances don't share a wide range of interests with me. For example, we might go to a movie but never bike together. And those who could go on the four-hour ride I'd like to do occasionally are still working. Now, I have all this time during the week, but no one to play with."

"So, it's a sad situation?"

"Not devastating. More a sense of missed opportunities."

A reflective silence descended. Finally, I commented quietly that retirement might be a time for some processing of the regrets of youth, now that we no longer had jobs to hide behind. Megan lowered her head and stared at me from the top of her eyes.

"Don't worry," I hastened to say, "I'm not going to ask you to confess your youthful indiscretions."

"What makes you think I had any?" she retorted. "I was very discreet."

❋　❋　❋

I'd been pondering how retirement is affected by the extent to which it is voluntary. I vaguely recalled reading that a critical factor for men was whether they felt they were leaving work on their own terms.

"Tell me," I asked Megan, "how it was that you decided to retire when you did. You went early, and I've assumed this was pretty much your choice. Was there actually more going on, complicating your situation?"

"Yes," she sighed, "It was partly push and partly pull. I started thinking about going at fifty-five because that was the earliest I'd be able to access my pension. I was tired of commuting and in a rut at work. I wondered about retiring and teaching a little yoga part-time. I talked with my bank and attended a workshop that my pension plan offers. The financial penalty for retiring before sixty was significant, so I decided fifty-five wasn't the right age for me.

"Fortunately, I was able to take on a work project that I was passionate about. Time passed, then I went to another retirement seminar about a year ago. I learned that the pension plan was going to be changing in ways that would disadvantage me if I stayed employed. The financial numbers were now working in my favour.

"Just as importantly, I wasn't happy at work. As the result of yet another reorganization, I'd recently been redeployed into a new department in a modified role, again dealing with employees rather than providing patient care. I felt it as a push out. I didn't care for my new manager, and that solidified my decision.

"It wasn't a nice feeling to sense I no longer had a spot in my workplace of twenty-five years. With no formal transition, I wandered over to my new department and said,

'I think I'm supposed to be here. Where do you want me to sit?' That wasn't much fun. The new department didn't know what to do with me for the first four or five months. My move was handled poorly, and that hurt me. Not only did I not want to be at work anymore, I didn't have to be."

"Big organizations and half-baked ideas from the top," I said. "Health care seems to have lots of them, all exacerbated by poor communication. An observation based on my non-existent expertise." Megan gently nodded her head in polite agreement, her shoulder-length brown hair swaying gently, but I felt uncomfortable even as I spoke. *Stay on task,* I told myself. *I'm supposed to be interviewing, not chatting idly. My opinions don't matter right now.*

"I'll stop pontificating," I attempted to get back on track, "so I can ask you about your planning. You clearly considered your finances carefully. The literature suggests that's the extent of most people's planning. You, though, seemed to do a good job of thinking about other aspects of retirement, about what your life would look like after you stopped working full-time."

"Thanks for the compliment," she said. "I accept it gratefully, all the more because I did indeed do a fair amount of thinking about my future. My idea was to retire in the spring, have a leisurely summer, and then reassess. Was I able to fill my time, or was I bored? Was I enjoying what I was doing, or did I want more? I'm still in that stage right now. Because work was a big part of my social life, I wanted to ensure I had enough part-time work for the short term, create some new social connections, find a new hobby or passion, and so on. That's still unfolding."

"Staying on the planning theme," I asked, "has anything

occurred that you didn't anticipate?"

Megan again took time to formulate a thoughtful response. "I didn't fully anticipate," she searched for words, "the changed ethos or tone of my life. I'm finding it strange right now. I'm feeling a bit that I don't know what to do or what's next. That's not bad or negative. It's just sitting and wondering what the coming months are going to look like."

Her voice became more animated. "I've noticed that even though I planned not to do much for six months, I'm not very good at doing little. I almost overcommit because that's what I've been used to doing. When I have big pieces of space, I feel I should be doing something. It's a carry-over from my previous life. I'm just starting to give myself permission to have a nap in the middle of the day or to sit and read a book all afternoon.

"Slowing down is not so easy. That's been one of the bigger challenges for me. I like to get out and about, but then I get exhausted. In fact, I got vertigo within two weeks of retiring. That was the universe telling me to get in balance because I was tired. If we don't listen to our body, our body will do it for us. It said to me, 'Enough. I'm laying you flat out for a while.'

"Looking back, vertigo was a positive thing to happen to me, even though being nauseous wasn't. I began taking things more slowly and watching what I was eating. That put me into a good place for moving forward. After years of working, commuting, and always moving, it was almost as if my body had to detox from these habits. You have to give yourself permission to slow down."

❋   ❋   ❋

"Let me ask how your self-image might be changing," I said. "It sounds like you're having a hard time letting go of your past identity as a doer, a worker, somebody who has to cram too much into the week. Are there other ways in which you might be grappling, if that's not too strong a word, with how you see yourself?"

"I want to be clear," Megan said, "that my occupation wasn't always my primary identity. I was a mom and didn't start working full-time until I was in my forties. I had connections not only through work but also through family. That was common for women of my generation with kids. It could be different for men."

I thought Megan might say more about gender, but she instead shrugged her shoulders and began talking about aging. "It's not just about leaving work. It's also about loss of your youth." I nodded as she continued. "Now you're a senior and viewed as elderly. I don't see myself as that, so maybe that's partly why I'm a little out of sorts. That active phase of my life is over. Now I'm entering the winter of my life. It's the last season, but I'm not ready to hang out at the senior's centre, even with active seniors. I want to be with people of all ages.

"I reconnected not so long ago with a group of people I've known for a long time. I was the youngest. Most were sixty-five to seventy. They spent their whole time—well, a lot of time—talking about their doctors' appointments, their MRIs, CT scans, medication, and how to get the cheapest travel health insurance. Three were walking with canes or had had hips and knees done.

"They were old. They had taken their careers very seriously, working long hours and doing nothing when they got home. This is where I can see how important it is to stay active. If you don't use it, you'll lose it for sure. They had a different philosophy than me about how to live one's life.

"It's finding my right niche. I don't want to hang out with people who can't go for a walk. Yet, there are some people my age running triathlons. I'm not in that category either."

I've heard other seniors complaining about getting stuck with old people, but I hadn't expected Megan to bring up this topic. She mentioned someone who, at age sixty, had said that she felt invisible. "I didn't understand at the time what she was saying. Now, I'm starting to get it because we live in a very youth-oriented society. The wisdom of the elder would be nice to reclaim. It's not valued and honoured in our society." By way of example, she described friends who hardly see their kids and grandkids. "It's not that there was a big blowout. It's more the kids thinking that they don't need their parents in their lives."

Megan put her elbows on the table and leaned her head into her upturned hands. She stared at me and said, "I'm definitely in a transition period, but it doesn't seem right to say that my identity is changing. I feel like the same person. You know, I have a retired friend who said she started going back and doing a lot of things she used to do in high school, but which she had let slide. She wasn't changing her identity. She was reclaiming it.

"I haven't played my clarinet for a decade, yet I know there's a community band I could now join. I used to love making music, but I gave it up when I got married. My creative side suffered in the workplace. It was a very left-brain type of place—structured, hierarchical, and procedure driven. I'd like to tap back into my creative side.

"That may be why I'm feeling a little out of sorts, not in a bad way. As I transition, there are bits of me I'm letting go of, but bits I'm trying to open up to. I'm inclined to think I'm not quite the same person as I was a year or two before retirement. Yet who I am fundamentally is unchanged. I've done a lot of unpeeling my layers over the past decade. I'm just trying to reconnect with parts of myself that got lost or buried."

The sounds of a car alarm in the next block distracted me as Megan said that she hadn't previously considered whether she is still the same person. "It's an interesting question, though. As I talk with you, these aha moments come along."

"That's been my experience with many of the life-journey interviews I've conducted for other projects," I said. "We typically live our lives in little pieces. Telling a big portion of your story to somebody else helps you see the forest and not only the trees. To see the broad contours and significant forces. And it doesn't seem to matter how ordinary a person's life has been. Something interesting and important always emerges."

✳   ✳   ✳

"I've been asking a lot of questions and shaping the conversation," I said. "Maybe other topics are also relevant, but it hasn't occurred to me to ask you about them. Are there other things you could mention that would help me better understand your past few months?"

I should have known better than to ask a closed question

where a simple "No" by way of response could end the discussion. Fortunately, Megan seemed to be enjoying the chance to talk, and she took a few moments to search for other observations to share with me.

"I suppose I started on the retirement journey with a positive outlook in that I had a good role model in my dad, who retired at fifty-seven. I saw him transition successfully. He had a good ten years of retirement before he got sick. That's not long. We don't know what's coming, even though we can try to mitigate health with our lifestyle. I want to enjoy some retirement time. Life is short."

Megan turned silent, her body language suggesting she was actively considering whether she wanted to add anything else. Finally, I said, "I'm increasingly coming to think that the notion of a transition period, perhaps in the year before retirement as well as in the year afterwards, is a key concept for planning and understanding feelings during these years. What are your thoughts about transitions?"

Better, I thought. That was a good, open-ended question.

"When people are retiring," she said carefully, "they need to be aware that their habitual patterns are going to change. Perhaps the detox might be to shed structure slowly. For example, set your alarm just a little later, then later again. Wean yourself off work gradually.

"I had reduced my work week to eighty percent during my last two years. That was a small adjustment. In retrospect, rather than using up all my remaining vacation in one block just before retiring, perhaps I should have used those days to shorten my work week gradually, moving from eighty percent to sixty and then forty. That might have been a better transition from a physical health point of view. A gradual transition out of work might have made my energy change feel less dramatic."

After a long pause, I smiled, "And now, the predictable question. Is there anything, as you look back, you would do differently?"

"I'm not so sure I would have predicted that question, but at least it's one that I've asked myself. Leading up to retirement, no. Afterwards, I should have stuck more to my guns about not doing too much. Just maintain the things I was already doing for the first six months. Just relax, breathe, and get into a routine. I still feel driven."

She hastened to add, "Before I give the impression that I'm too much of a Type A personality, you need to know that I've been stopping to smell a few roses as I make my way to yet one more activity. And combining that with a bit of adventure. For example, I've been using transit more often, learning the system, since I have the time and, at some point, driving may not be an option for me. I've explored new places, taking different bus routes or getting off early and walking the last part in order to soak up the atmosphere of new neighbourhoods."

Now it was Megan's turn to smile at me. "That part about walking is a segue. I've really enjoyed talking, but I have to be on my way. Was anything I said close to what you were looking for?" She placed her left hand on the table as she gently rose from her seat, twisting to reach her purse's shoulder strap from the chair back.

"You bet," I nodded. "That was great. And I really enjoyed listening."

BRONWYN

"Bronwyn," I announced, "I've been reading about the potential losses that worry some people when they think about retiring. There's loss of status and identity from their job, of course. Reduced income, less intellectual stimulation, loss of daily structure, less social contact, and so on. Maybe even loss of meaning to their life in extreme cases. It's all good stuff, but it's getting repetitive. Were you afraid of losing anything that might not be so predictable?"

Bronwyn leaned forward in her chair, assessed me carefully, and slightly turned up the corners of her mouth. "I guess this means my interview has started? You don't waste any time with preliminaries, do you?"

Her words took me back. "Sorry for being so abrupt," I hastily replied. "I guess I got a little carried away. Let's hold that question, and I'll try to start properly."

"No, it's okay. I'm just giving you a hard time. You provided enough of an introduction when we arranged a time to meet. Just give me a moment to think."

Bronwyn stared vacantly over my right shoulder while she sipped her tea. The blue and green pattern on the earthenware mug was angular and abstract, but it nonetheless managed to suggest something organic.

"How about this?" she finally said. "I used to work mainly with men, and I enjoyed them. I was aware that once I retired, my circle would become heavily female. I was a bit concerned because men have different perspectives and ways of being. They talk about different things. Of course, you interact with them differently in a professional setting than you do outside of work."

"Yes," I said, "that's a different twist on social interaction that I've not heard before. How big a deal was it for you?"

"Medium, at most. While I was reluctant to give up the male contact, I certainly wasn't going to let it hold me back. Life always involves trade-offs."

"Would I be pushing my luck if I asked whether you had anything else out of the ordinary?"

"Unusual in what way?"

"Same topic. Concern about losing something that isn't so predictable."

She shook her head. "It was hard enough coming up with the male thing. So, no, I don't think I have any quirky regrets."

"Fair enough. Now, let me go back and ease into this interview. You retired early from your job, so how about describing the process by which you decided when you wanted to leave?"

"That's a good way for me to start. It's easier for me to tell you about things in the sequence they occurred, rather than bouncing around randomly from topic to topic." Bronwyn took one more sip and then launched in.

"I wanted to retire before age sixty, and I achieved that

by one week. I had two reasons for retiring early. One driver was that my father had died at age sixty-one and didn't have a retirement. I know that health is never guaranteed, and I wanted a whirl at a good retirement. I wasn't paranoid about health issues, but they were a consideration in the back of my mind.

"The bigger factor was that I had achieved a sense of fulfillment. I had worked full-time for thirty-eight years, mostly in the public sector but also in a non-profit. In thinking how my life might unfold, I never envisioned a run that long and steady. I also had a good diversity of work experiences that I was proud of—some real high points, along with some tough times as well. I wanted to go while I was still enthusiastic. When you get to the point where you think you've been around a mulberry bush four or five times already, I fretted that my attitude might deteriorate to the point where I was affecting other people."

"Leaving on a high point was important to you?" I summarized.

"Yes. I had a good reputation and wanted to be remembered that way. My workplace was volatile, and the possibility of ending on a low note was quite real. It's better having people begging you to stay than helping you out the door."

I wondered if it was hard as the exit day approached.

"No. In the months before retirement, I was fairly calm because I had been thinking for several years as to what my date might be. I didn't have anything firmly in mind until I was in a particular monthly meeting that drove me nuts. I vividly remember thinking, 'That's it. I'm going one year from now.' That decision brought me great joy in the subsequent monthly meetings.

"I could have gone at age fifty-five," she concluded, "but I never gave it serious thought. I absolutely could not envision staying until sixty-five."

A comfortable silence hung for a few moments. While Bronwyn pushed her glasses higher on her nose, a distant train whistle joined the chorus of nearby birds.

"What type of planning or thinking did you do as to what your life might be like after you retired?" I asked. "I mean, thoughts while you were still working."

"I figured retirement would have at least two stages. I wanted to begin with a whole year of no commitments. I'm good at commitments, and I didn't want to exchange one kind of busyness for another kind of busyness.

"Twenty or so years ago, a whole group of us were laid off when our organization went through a major overhaul. I had been thinking at that time that it might be nice to take a sabbatical year, perhaps to travel. However, I ended up landing a new job quite quickly, so the sabbatical never came to be.

"In my first retirement year, I wanted to take the time and be intentional about what my new lifestyle would be. I did intend to volunteer, but not until I was ready to have regular commitments again. I was aware that my church activity could become all-consuming. I knew I needed to be intentional if I didn't want to get sucked in—which I didn't.

"Of course, I didn't see everything as rosy and wonderful. Because I live alone, I was aware that when I was no longer busy around people all day, it might become problematic. I wasn't sure. When you're really busy and working full-time, your home is a sanctuary. When that busyness lessens, there's less need to withdraw and have quiet time.

"Most of the books in the library about retirement planning," I said, "concern financial planning. Were you anxious about money?"

"No, not at all. I'm aware that not everybody can say that. Health and finances were not issues for me, which they could easily have been."

"How emotional were your last days or weeks at work?" I inquired for a second time, hoping I might elicit more drama.

"I didn't have any strong emotions as the time approached. I'd done enough processing as I made the decision, completed the paperwork, and told people. When the day came, I had been in a different headspace for quite some time. I also had two small trips and one big one planned for the coming months—something to look forward to immediately, as opposed to just looking back.

"On retirement day, a friend in another department took me for a drink since my retirement party was going to be held a couple of weeks later. She offered to walk out of the building with me for the last time, and I did get a bit choked up. Jumping ahead in my story, a year later, after having done some part-time work for the same organization, I couldn't get out the door fast enough. Even though my director wanted me to come in the next day and I'd had a positive experience, I just said no and left."

"I take it then," I surmised, "that you saw retirement more as stepping into an opportunity than as a loss?"

"Absolutely as an opportunity. I've never been defined by my job, although it may have been a lot of my identity in other people's eyes. I was never so wedded to my career that

I thought that leaving would be an issue for me. There were so many other things that I would have preferred to have been doing while I was employed. And I didn't need more money in order to maintain my modest lifestyle."

Bronwyn waited patiently while I finished scribbling my notes. I'd learned from interviews I'd conducted for other projects that these pauses could be valuable processing times for my interviewees. Sometimes, overlooked points or new insights emerged, but that wasn't the case this time.

❄   ❄   ❄

"Let's shift now," I said, "to the early days of your retirement." I reiterated the purpose of my project, emphasizing that social networks or, at least, the challenge of maintaining social contact is different for singles than couples. "Given this background, to what extent were you intentional about meeting with people, and was loneliness ever an issue?"

Bronwyn squirmed a little. "Good topic, but it's a big one. I'll try to focus on what arose because of retirement and wasn't just a reflection of my personal situation."

After a few moments, she said slowly, "It was a challenge living alone and no longer being busy around other people five days a week. I had few people with whom I could have more than a superficial conversation. It's not that when you're at work or in your regular routines that you're having heart-to-hearts every day, but it was different once I retired. As coworkers, we continually knew what was going on in at least parts of each other's lives.

"I also live in a rental building in a large city, and I have no sense of neighbourhood. That doesn't mean I'm not friendly to the people I see in the hallway, but I usually don't see anyone there. And once again, it ends up being superficial conversation. It's not like a single-family neighbourhood where people spend time in their yards and have long talks over the fence with people with whom they have a history. Vancouver is known for not being friendly, so my experience wasn't unusual. Loneliness and a lack of community are broader societal issues."

"What about people who weren't close friends but who were more than casual acquaintances?" I probed.

"On the positive side, it was gratifying when such people were pleased to see me again or made the effort to stay in touch. Nevertheless, I found that connecting with them only occasionally took energy. So much of the conversation was catching up, explaining what I'd been doing or inquiring about the other person. They were pleasant encounters, but more backwards-looking than forward-focused. Kind of one-shot deals.

"The backdrop to this is that I have a small extended family. We get along well, but most are independent and want less frequent contact than I do. This left me feeling a little isolated, and that unless I initiated gatherings, they wouldn't happen. My relatives wouldn't share this perception, but that's how it felt to me."

I know that family dynamics are important, but this wasn't a subject I wanted to explore because I feared it could take on a life of its own, leading me far from the topic of retirement. I promptly changed the subject. "What were some of the first joys that came from not working?"

Bronwyn flashed another of her smiles that lights up the room. "Not setting the alarm clock, not being conscientious about bedtime, and especially lingering over coffee on Monday mornings. Some people might say there was a little gloating, but I wouldn't.

"Another aspect of freedom from schedules was being able to shop, or drive, or ski in the daytime, midweek. It was an eye-opener. I'd never seen so many preschoolers and babies in my life.

"Maybe my escape from schedules was a little too extreme. I had so many nights of long sleep that I mildly wondered if something was wrong with me. And then I found it hard to be on time, even for a midmorning coffee date or lunch at noon. I had spent so much of my life watching the clock that I stopped watching it, sometimes to my detriment. It's embarrassing when you're retired and can't be on time."

"Seriously?" I asked. "I've never known you to be late."

"I kid you not," she replied.

I returned my gaze to my notepad and waited for whatever might surface next.

"It was just nice to have time to do things at leisure, even at home," Bronwyn said. "Like organizing my walk-in locker and playing the piano for a change. More time for my stamp and photo collections, having a regular morning devotional time. And having time to do ordinary fitness things outside the home, such as walking more, attending fitness classes regularly, and upgrading my bike." Her voice trailed off.

Eventually, I asked if she felt much of an identity change in that first half year.

"Yes and no," she replied. "Although I wasn't sixty-five, I was a senior in the sense that I was a pensioner. I don't identify with the term senior—am I really in that category? How did I get here?—but I'm happy to take advantage of it to get a cheap deal or preferential treatment. It's kind of a funny feeling, like I'm fraudulently taking advantage of society.

"I've finally gotten over being indignant when somebody offers me a seat on the bus based solely on my hair colour, especially when I've just been cross-country skiing or to a cardio class. Now, I'm at the point where I think it's good to reward them for being polite. Sometimes, I have packages, and I am actually glad to take their seat. So, I'm over that part."

"Have any Boy Scouts tried to help little old lady Bronwyn across the street?" I asked with as much innocence I could muster. She ignored me.

"Maybe there's something bigger here," she mused, "in terms of identity. I felt people were trying to pigeonhole me far too frequently." Seeing my perplexed expression, she explained, "After I retired, I was unexpectedly asked to return to work on contract a couple of days per week. I hadn't given that possibility a second thought, but when it came along, it proved to be a helpful personal transition. By this time, I was an outsider to the organization, but an insider in that I still knew everybody and all the projects. My former colleagues were glad to see me. I was a safe person with whom they felt they could share their issues and, occasionally, even vent. I enjoyed it, but it took energy. I felt I was being paid more to be a listening post than to be productive. Kind of strange, but a good way of winding down and bringing closure to my former role.

"Anyhow, what all this has to do with identity was that

people were confused about my employment status. I got tired of explaining to people who were out of date with me and especially to people who should have known. Sometimes people were just trying to be nice and make conversation but didn't know what else to say. It was annoying, nevertheless.

"Plus, I didn't know how long the contract work would carry on, so it was hard to be clear about an ambiguous arrangement that was working well for all the concerned parties. After a year of this, I decided it's better to be retired or not retired, rather than sort of retired.

"I'm afraid I'm sounding like I'm whining or ungrateful. That's not the case at all. It was nice to be wanted. It was a wonderful way to wind down my working life, and I valued it. I got lots of hugs whenever I showed up, which I hadn't expected."

I sensed a broader issue here, but couldn't quite name it. "What you're saying is resonating with me, but I'm having a hard time figuring out how. Maybe that it's easier for us to navigate when the people we meet fit in neat categories. Is anything along these lines relevant to your retirement experiences?"

Bronwyn pursed her lips. She tipped her mug and peered into it. "Maybe. Here's a roundabout response. You can decide if it applies.

"I got annoyed when people asked me what I was up to now or how I spent my time. It felt like I had to justify myself. I understood the question was usually well intended, but I sometimes received it as judgmental, or it was asked because the other person feared they wouldn't know what to do if they were in my shoes. I hope I never ask other people those questions and especially not if they're keeping busy. The best answer I could give was that I was trying to *be* and not *do*. That gave them something a little different to think about!"

We sat in more silence. I eventually asked if, looking back after four or six months, Bronwyn had felt her retirement preparations had been realistic and sufficient.

"For sure, financially." She said she purposely hadn't touched any of her investments because she wanted to see if her pension would support her lifestyle, which really didn't change much. "Just a greater need for casual, outdoor clothes. The pension proved totally adequate.

"Overall, I must have prepared well because I didn't encounter any bumps in the road. Everything just proceeded ordinarily."

"So, in a nutshell," I suggested, "your transition into retirement was gentle."

"Yes. I was very happy for six months. It was like a honeymoon period. You get to do these things, try these things. Everybody knows it's a new phase for you. I feel like I sailed through it."

﹡   ﹡   ﹡

I looked up. "Do I detect some ominous foreshadowing here? Honeymoons eventually end."

"Maybe not ominous, but I was surprised that the next six months were harder. It was only then that it dawned on me that I was truly building a new lifestyle."

"In what ways?"

'You might laugh," she said, "but shaking the work ethic

has been harder than I expected."

My body language must have communicated something I hadn't intended, because Bronwyn immediately began explaining herself. "I haven't completely recovered from the niggling sense that I should be doing something. Then I realize there's absolutely nothing I have to do today. It's quite lovely, but I look forward to not having the buried expectation that there's something left to do. That comes from having been busy for so long. Having the freedom to choose is taking more getting used to than I expected.

"And speaking of time, it can be feast or famine. Everything happens and then nothing does. When I was working, I was always apportioning my time—there was never enough—and things tended to be spread out more evenly."

I suspected that scheduling time with friends, at least with some friends, doesn't necessarily become easier in retirement. Bronwyn confirmed this, without me having to ask.

"I discovered there were people I didn't want to spend more time with. With the people I did want to see, it became a scheduling exercise. In what areas did we share interests, and when were they available to do them? Did we have the same budget? For example, did they always want to go for supper before a show or never?

At times, I felt like I was back at work doing team management. It never totally discouraged me from making the effort, but it caused me to consider whether I really wanted to try that hard. I eventually began watching for people who responded well or reciprocated and also took some initiative."

I stopped writing and made a comment about Megan. "I was talking to a retiree who said that some of her friends from her working days were more convenient habits than soulmates. She found that spending more time with them now was sucking the life out of her." I paused. "Maybe she didn't express it quite that strongly."

"Maybe she did," Bronwyn countered. "I absolutely get it. Then you have to make a decision as to whether this is a role that you're willing to play for them, and that maybe it's all for them, or do you need to be nurtured yourself? I find myself asking how important it is to have a big circle. Perhaps if you have two or three good friendships, that more than balances having many people on your periphery.

"Travelling is one of the areas where I feel this tension most profoundly. It's lovely to have the time and interest and money to travel, but I don't have obvious companions. It does make me a little anxious about knowing who wants to do what, when, and at what cost. I'm not big on travelling alone, even in a group tour.

"Incidentally," she barked, "don't ask me where I'm off to next or what places are still on my list. I'm adamantly against bucket lists—I think it's such a first-world privilege—and I try to cherish each trip as it happens, instead of treating it like one more item to check off."

I glanced at my watch, relieved that we hadn't been talking for as long as I thought. I could ask some more questions. "You've been speaking about time and friends. How are you finding it now that you have time for all sorts of activities in addition to time for friends?"

"Obviously, it's nice. But strangely, being able to do anything at anytime became wearing. It takes energy to try new things. You find out some are good, but some are not appealing. That tired me sometimes."

"But isn't that a welcome tiredness, a happy fatigue?"

"When things go well, yes. But in this experimenting stage, not everything does." She continued more pensively, "There were things in the first six months that I definitely want to continue, but other things gave me pause. I realized that I needed to be very intentional because certain things are not within my control. For example, the two elderly relatives I could now support more fully had died. Another example is perhaps the friendship issue we just talked about. I had lots of time now for friends, but discovered there were people who I didn't want to see all that often."

I took advantage of the slower pace to stretch and wiggle in my chair. When I'm taking notes, I tend to hunch too much.

"I'm again hearing the theme you alluded to at the beginning." I observed, "about retirement having stages. It seems that part of this is some trial and error until you find your groove."

Bronwyn considered this remark for a while, slowly nodding her head. "Yes. My intention to find a new volunteer activity took three tries. Although I didn't have my heart set on my first two ideas, I was still quite interested in each. By the time the third one came along, I recognized it as a good fit. Finally. I was glad it had finally come.

"Comically, I'm volunteering back at a place I used to work many years ago, although in a completely different role. Somebody asked if I might develop PTSD from returning there. I actually did think about the wisdom of returning, but the organizational turmoil has long since passed. The past dysfunction had nothing to do with me personally. As a volunteer now, I don't feel any pressure or have bad associations."

The reference to former workplaces reminded me that I had a badminton game to get to that afternoon, located in a gym across the street from where I had once worked. It was time to begin wrapping up with Bronwyn.

"Now the big question," I said, catching Bronwyn's attention. "In retrospect, with your twenty-twenty vision, do you wish you had done anything differently?"

"Good question," she acknowledged. "I think I've avoided facing it." She sat silently for half a minute. "No, I don't believe I would." She tilted her head. "I suppose I could have worked part-time slightly longer into my first year of retirement, but I think the partnership would have become a less happy one as time passed. It could have fizzled out. I'm glad I went at a high point."

"You're talking about a high point again."

She smiled.

"Are your emotional fluctuations any different now that you're retired? I mean week to week, not at any particular moment."

Bronwyn again considered my question carefully before answering, "I don't think I'm any different or that I fluctuate all that much. I'm happy to be retired. My timing was right. I have the privilege of a retirement that's adequately funded. I'm aware my health status can change in a second, so I try to appreciate what I have now. I'd say I'm happily retired."

GILLIAN

I regretted that Gillian didn't meet my retirement criterion because she seemed a fascinating person. I already knew she had done a stint of nursing in the Arctic and volunteered here in the south at a hospice. An energetic and gregarious person, she had, among other things, organized recreational outings for women in the Red Hat Society and helped to train assistance dogs. I wanted to learn what made her tick, but the inconvenient truth was that she had been married when she retired.

"Only the first time," she corrected me. "So, you could include my story if you want."

"The first time?"

"Yes, I was single the second time."

"Was that the last time you retired?"

"Yes. At least, I think so. I'm not planning to return to work yet again."

My curiosity and disappointment growing, I sighed. "I'd love to include you, but it's that initial transition into retirement and what happened afterwards that matter. You're telling me you were married when your retirement saga began. Whatever the circumstances of your marriage, you didn't enter retirement all by yourself."

Gillian flatly disagreed. "Yes, I did. I was emotionally single."

Emotionally single. Now there was a variation I hadn't taken into account.

She continued, "I had tried therapy and did everything I could think of to make our relationship work. Nothing helped. Finally, I simply deadened myself as a coping strategy."

"But surely your husband was in some way part of your decision-making about retirement?" I asked, trying to understand her adamant viewpoint.

"No. Neither did my own wishes enter the picture. I had to retire of necessity. It wasn't a choice." She gazed at me intently. "You can't get much more alone than being unconnected to even yourself."

I had to concede that she had a point. I revised my thinking about what it means to be single.

❋ ❋ ❋

"My two retirements," Gillian began, "will make a lot more sense if I give you some history about my back injury, decades earlier." She described how that injury had kept her away from work for almost five years and brought her to an existential turning point. "After my original injury, I couldn't do anything, not even lift a carton of milk from the fridge or open the sliding door to the patio. If I went out in the morning, I had to forget the remainder of the day. If I was going out in the evening, I had to rest up all day.

"My health problems led to a big identity crisis. Who was I, and what was my purpose in life? I'm not Nurse, I thought. I can hardly be Wife in this crummy marriage. I can't even be Housekeeper with this injury. Plus, I had to give up my marathon running, which had taken a huge amount of time and been a big part of my social life. Working full-time, marathoning, and going to the gym five days a week all disappeared in a hurry. So now, I wasn't Athlete, or Nurse. Who was I? I found out I could be Student. That was good. That's why I became over-educated."

Gillian first returned to school because life had become unbearably boring when she was off work. Her program led to a nursing specialization in neo-natal intensive care. "I thought that if I could no longer care for big people, maybe I could look after tiny babies. That didn't work out, though, because of the way I had to twist and bend in the nursery." Then, she upgraded her RN diploma from a hospital nursing school to a bachelor's degree from a university.

When she graduated from these studies, Gillian still wasn't sufficiently healthy to return to nursing. She continued as a student, completing a master's degree from an American university. "Now, I was ready and wanting to return to work, but I couldn't find a job in my new field because the States were way ahead of Canada in using clinical nurse specialists. Canada now has those types of jobs, but I was before my time."

Reluctantly, Gillian changed the focus of her practice from adventure nursing, flying to oil rigs and bush camps, to a less physically demanding psychosocial role. "I used to work in wild places and do outlandish stuff. Now, I faced a huge shift in my career." She found a part-time position and never again held a full-time job. "But," she added with a sideways glance, "I often worked more than full-time hours because I could. I was in a psychiatric unit, and the job was fairly sedentary. I kept working because I didn't want to be at home. Work, work, and more work."

✻   ✻   ✻

Gillian had chosen to sit at my dining-room table on a hard, straight chair rather than lounge on the sofa. She had entered the room with a slightly stiff gait and lowered herself carefully to her seat. I glanced at her, wondering if I should ask whether she was still comfortable, but everything seemed normal. I remained silent.

"Now, you know enough to understand my first retirement," she said. "I had to retire from nursing because of my back. It was a medical issue. That was really hard, giving up my occupation."

"Did you come to that decision yourself, or did somebody else tell you to leave?"

She waggled her head from side to side. "A bit of both, I think."

"You'll have to explain that to me."

"It was a prolonged process. I've told you about returning to school for a number of years. Well, our collective agreement ensured my position would be held for me for two years while I was off. I was physically unable to return after two years, so my job was posted and somebody else filled it. I was now unemployed, and there weren't a lot of nursing jobs I was physically capable of doing. I worried I was being forced involuntarily into a very early retirement.

"I kept searching, though, and eventually found a position in mental health and addictions as an injection nurse, shooting people up with antipsychotics all day long. With previous experience in this field, I really enjoyed the role, both my colleagues and the clients. This was the perfect job for me to coast through my remaining work years. But then my back acted up, again. When I started dragging my leg behind me, I asked for six weeks off, but my supervisor said she was going to post my job. 'No, no,' I pleaded, 'just give me a couple of weeks. I'll be fine.' Well, a couple of weeks later, I still couldn't return to work, and I reluctantly had to let that job go."

I asked if this was when she formally retired, giving up any hope or intention of nursing again. "Yes," she replied, she had resigned herself to the inevitable.

"Was leaving every bit as much about losing a profession as losing income or filling your time?"

"Definitely, but this time differed from my other times off work in that I had finally realized I had been far too wrapped up in my nursing identity. I now recognized that I needed a new lifestyle. At one point, I had four part-time nursing jobs all at once. I was a total workaholic. People would ask, 'What do you do?' and I'd say, 'I'm a nurse.' That's all I could say. Now my answer is, 'I do this, and this, and this.' But I had to make a conscious effort to change."

"Okay," I said, "I've enjoyed hearing everything you've told me, but now we're finally at the relevant part of your story, namely your first year of retirement."

"Yes." Gillian smiled. "I did my best to prolong the tension before my big reveal." She studied her watch. "Maybe I've run out of time, and you'll have to wait until another day to find out what happened."

"Nice try. Get on with it." I put on my sternest face but to no effect. Gillian continued to smirk defiantly at me, then relented.

"I started retirement married, but emotionally single. From a practical point of view, I was well set up. I had a place to live, after all. But I was thinking hard about leaving my marriage. If I came to that decision, there were certain things I wanted to have in place. Like having some sort of a job with benefits."

"If you had been happily married, do you think you would have been content to remain retired?"

"Probably not. Even if my family life had been good, I still would have found it monotonous. Boredom was why I returned to school so quickly. I hurt my back at the end of May, and by September, I was in school. I have to be doing something because I don't entertain myself very well. I discovered I liked going to school, and I was good at it.

"The reality was that I didn't want to be at home because of the state of my marriage. After a couple of months, I searched online for something I could do. I found a little job in a music school that was literally two blocks up the road from where I lived."

As we talked, I realized Gillian had worked at the music school my daughters attended several years prior. I mentioned that I used to look forward to sitting with my eldest in the four- and five-year-old class because the instructor, a retired kindergarten teacher, was the most skilful instructor I had ever observed. Plus, she had improved my musical ear, albeit that I'm still largely tone-deaf. But I digress.

Gillian worked two days a week as a cashier-receptionist.

"I got along famously," she said, "and became close friends with the owner and his family. I had a good musical background, and everything was great. The job provided some structure to my week in addition to my three volunteer activities. I was learning new stuff that had nothing to do with nursing.

"Best of all, it was a very social job. I got to know so many people—I still get phone calls from some of the piano moms. There were tears when I left, and I wasn't the only one crying. To this day, five to ten years later, kids will come up to me and say, 'Hey, you're the piano lady.'"

I nodded in recognition. My father had been a high-school teacher. I recalled many a conversation with a former student where Dad's use of certain phrases signalled to the family whether he could remember the student or not. Regardless, the conversations were amiable; one of the delayed perks for educators that help offset the numerous daily challenges they face.

"But you eventually left this job," I prompted.

"After four years, a few people started to get on my nerves, and I began wondering if this indicated it was time to finish this chapter of my life. One of the teachers begged me not to leave, so I stayed an additional year. I probably shouldn't have. By the time I left, I was so ready to exit, despite loving many aspects of the job. I did have a blow-up with one particular teacher, although we're cordial when we encounter each other now."

"This was when you retired for good?"

"Yes."

"How was it this time?"

"While at the music school, I left my husband. I was

now single, but I had built a life that wasn't just nursing. That was so very healthy, and I was glad I had made a deliberate effort to broaden. I realized I needed other things in my life so that I wouldn't be bored when I wasn't working. Now, I'm one of those retirees who says, 'How did I ever find time to work?' Retirement the second time round was different."

"You make it sound easy, but on top of retirement, you were also dealing with a recent divorce. That seems to me to be a lot to cope with."

Gillian shrugged. "It wasn't such a big deal. Although single, I had cultivated a fabulous circle of friends. A deep circle of supportive friends who helped me through both my divorce and second retirement."

✻   ✻   ✻

It seemed she had nothing more to say, yet I struggled to accept that things had been so uneventful in the end. I asked why she thought her second retirement had been smooth when the previous decade—better make that plural—had been full of drama. It took a while for her to work through the reasons and then find words to articulate them. They had to do with the conditions of departure.

"The first time round, I didn't want to go. The second time, I was ready. It was me who made the decision, and it worked well. I still stay in touch with the school, but I have never regretted leaving. The transition wasn't difficult because I was already volunteering, had friends outside of work, and wanted to travel. Plus, it was only a part-time job that I was leaving."

"I'm starting to understand. I've heard elsewhere that intentional preparation for life after work, and leaving on your own terms, are hugely helpful in getting off to a good start in retirement. Those seem to be important reasons for the differences between your two retirements."

Gillian thought for a moment and then bobbed in agreement. I caught her attention again, a moment later, when I mentioned my curiosity about a topic she hadn't mentioned, but which is front and centre for so many retirees.

"What topic?"

"Finances."

"What about finances?"

"Will my monthly income be high enough? Will I be okay in the long run? These can be gigantic issues for people whose marriage ends later in life."

"Fortunately, not for me. I'm a saver, and I'd always paid attention to my money, so financial planning for retirement was just more of the same. In fact, I went to my first financial planning seminar when I was still in my twenties because I have this huge fear of running out of money. I don't know where that anxiety comes from because, despite a modest upbringing, I never wanted for anything, and I made good money as a nurse."

Once again, Gillian had surprised me with her response. Our conversation seemed to be reaching a natural conclusion. I remarked that she differed from people who had worked more or less full-time in the same occupation and then came to an abrupt stop when they retired. She had experienced a few disruptions in her life, with some periods off work and then returning to part-time jobs. In some ways, leaving the workforce was a slow process over many years, rather than a single event.

Gillian agreed with this summary, picking up the theme of loss. "When I had to stop running, that was hard for me. Running had been such a huge part of my social life. Then not going to work, I felt a big sense of loss. I've had several losses along the way, as opposed to one big grieving at age sixty-five. I also learned to be resilient, to face up to challenges, perhaps not overcoming them, but figuring out how to accommodate or work around them. Life is by no means perfect for me, but I find myself in a pretty good place at the moment." She added reflectively, "For which I'm grateful. My life right now could easily have been unpleasant."

STYMIED

Despite a promising start with three great interviews, my project had slowed to a standstill. All those retired people I knew were turning out to consist mainly of couples—not the demographic I wanted to reach—and women. Males who were single when they retired seemed to be an extinct species. I asked a few friends if they had contact with such unattached men. After long pauses, I usually heard, "Hmmm, good question. Nobody's coming to mind, but there must be some." *Yes*, I thought, *there must be some, but where are they?* In witness protection programs?

Rather than resorting to dating websites and posters on street lamps as a recruitment strategy, I decided to buy some time by browsing my local library. It's a small branch, and I suspected it might be less informative than the Internet, but libraries have a way of occasionally providing gems. And perhaps some interviewable guys would materialize in the interim.

The few books on topics other than financial planning mainly offered sound but boring advice, not descriptions of actual experiences. *Oh well, I tried,* I consoled myself.

Turning to the Internet, the first website I visited discussed a topic that was new to me, namely retiree guilt, a counterpart to survivor's guilt. As I browsed the postings, the comments came mostly from armed service and public safety personnel whose occupations had provided them with the opportunity to retire in their late forties or mid fifties. This explained why the contributors were encountering such digs as, "It must be nice to play all day while the rest of us are trapped at work." Understandable, but certainly special cases, so back to the library I ambled, this time to another branch.

I met with more success the second time round. One book talked specifically about men, asserting that retirement is one of the most complicated transitions many will ever navigate—not as hard, granted, as losing a partner, but challenging nonetheless. It claimed that one third of male retirees struggle in adjusting to retirement, despite often having a supportive spouse. The good news was that the strain is typically short-term, and most eventually adjust, with many thriving.

Another book described a study of adult development. It found that four elements were especially important in forging an agreeable retirement: making friends and strengthening social networks, playing and doing things that bring you pleasure, being creative regardless of your skill level, and continually learning new things. I gathered that it's not enough simply to keep busy doing the same old things. Rather, one needs also to evolve continually.

Perhaps they're not essential, but I'm inclined to think two other factors are also important for the happiness of seniors: contributing in some way to the well-being of others and staying physically fit. In any event, my daughter laughed as I burdened her with my latest insights from the library, especially about acquiring new interests. "A group of us at work were talking about parents who had divorced later in life," she began. She works in a newish IT company, where the staff is young and caregiving does not yet dominate conversations about parents. "Several parents had gone on to do things that their children never expected."

"For example?"

"One mom bought an RV and spent the first year of her retirement toodling around North America all by herself, although she met people along the way and sometimes connected with them again. Then she moved to a new city where one of her kids lived, sold her RV, bought a condo, and joined a quilting group. Nobody saw those activities coming. One of the dads walked the Camino de Santiago across northern Spain and published a book. On a different topic, not about the Camino."

I pondered the significance of these examples for retirees launching solo. Even though the single life has its challenges, not having to negotiate and compromise with a partner can make it easier to try out new roles and identities. The downside, of course, is that you don't have a companion encouraging you to dream nor a helpmate for realizing those dreams.

❋ ❋ ❋

I brought the beginning of this chapter to my Thursday morning writers' group. The city's recreation department offers this program to a wonderfully diverse set of a dozen individuals, some of whom return year after year while others come and go. If I wanted advice about how to reach into the community in search of elusive single, male retirees, this seemed a promising source.

As was our custom, I read my draft aloud while the others followed on their printed copies, occasionally scribbling in the margin or underlining a phrase. When I finished, I said, "So, in addition to your usual feedback about my writing technique, I'd also appreciate your thoughts as to how I might recruit more subjects to interview."

Justin, the group's facilitator and an editor by profession, presided at the head of the table in our spacious seminar room. "Are you nuts?" He glared at me. "We're here to critique each other's writing, not discuss research methodology. Get with the program."

I clenched my lips and met his gaze. *That's a fine example of small-mindedness*, I fumed, while deliberating whether to challenge his pronouncement. It might not hurt him, or the group for that matter, to colour outside the lines on occasion.

"Relax, just kidding," he said. I resumed breathing, sheepishly shaking my head. I always fall for his ruses. "Okay, folks, who has something helpful for Bob? In particular, does anybody know one of those single, male retirees? Or are they in such short supply that this is classified information, to be shared only with the most trusted of widows who happen to be on the prowl?"

I thrust my hand in my pocket, fumbling to retrieve my aluminum voice recorder and switch it on. I glanced around the room as I pushed it towards the centre of the laminate table. "Would it bother anybody if I record your comments? I don't want to miss anything."

"Just as long as you don't post it," came one reply.

"Not the slightest chance."

"If you do, you'll appear as a thinly disguised villain in every piece of fiction I ever publish."

"As if I don't already. In all two pieces, that is, that you've ever published."

Justin intervened to end the banter and steered the discussion back on track. My plea for ideas unleashed a flood of suggestions, some of which even helped me. Here's a sample of the conversation:

—You should join one of the city's senior centres. Hundreds of people belong to them, and it would be easy to chat there over coffee.

—But he's not sixty-five yet, so he can't join a centre. Or are you?

—No, no. You only have to be fifty. The centres are happening places, so they offer program for zoomers in addition to the frail and declining crowd.

—Maybe you'd encounter more guys if you played hockey or soccer. Let's face it, males are under-represented in our writing circles.

—Wouldn't guys have dropped out of those activities by retirement age?

—Not necessarily. Think about old-timer hockey.

—Say, another good sport might be pickleball. It's growing like mad, a soft landing for all the tennis players who have developed joint problems. Lots of retirees there.

—I've been thinking about teachers. Their two-month

break each summer is like a practice run for retirement. I wonder if they have different reactions than the rest of us when they finally call it a day?

—Don't forget about health care workers. Some of those unions have negotiated sweet contracts where long-serving employees get just about as much time off as teachers, plus big money on stat holidays.

—Now, don't start whining. We've already heard your rants about those collective agreements.

—It's one thing to give Bob ideas about where to find his target guys, but it's another to get them to talk about their feelings. At the risk of stereotyping, most guys aren't exactly socialized into being self-aware and reflective.

—I don't know if clamming up is all that gender specific. My daughter retired early to escape an unhappy job, and I worried how she'd do because she's a pretty quiet person. She took some classes to fill her time and would probably have lots to say that would interest Bob. I'll ask her if she'd be willing to be interviewed, but I expect she'll say no. That's based on her personality, not her gender.

* * *

Having journeyed to a federal government office in downtown Vancouver to replace a slightly water-damaged passport, I took the opportunity afterwards to visit the main library branch. There I found Robert Weiss's 2005 book, *The Experience of Retirement,* a summary for the general public of an academic study that included many interviews

with retirees. Weiss, a retired professor of sociology and ger-
ontology, hadn't focused on a particular demographic or on
the start of retirement the way I was, and he presented his
findings more thematically than in narrative form, but the
book was chock full of quotes and references to real people.
This was my kind of study, and it immediately resonated
with me.

In fact, I was hooked, even before the opening sentence,
by the foreword written by another professor, David Ekerdt.
I especially liked Ekerdt's paragraph encapsulating the
ambivalence of retirement:

> They contemplate retirement with hope and
> apprehension, want leisure but are still invested
> in work, and cherish the absence of stress and
> responsibility but miss the opportunity for
> achievement. Retirees have the sweet freedom
> of nothing special to do, but having nothing
> special to do likewise makes one socially mar-
> ginal. Relief from the interpersonal obligations
> of the workplace also means fewer people with
> whom to exchange favors or information.

One of Weiss's chapters considered all the reasons why
people retire, summarizing them in two broad categories.
One set of reasons has to do with the retiree's personal
circumstances and desires: some people are attracted by
the prospect of having more time for leisure, discretionary
activities, and family, while other retirees are constrained by
an aging body or illness. The other set of reasons arise from
the workplace itself. Sometimes, the job or other employees
are unpleasant, and the retiree simply wants to leave the

situation. Sometimes, the employer nudges or pushes the individual out, or the amount of work is reduced, and retirement seems preferable to unemployment and job hunting.

As I browsed the pages, I learned that orderly retirements, that is, ones with early planning and a predictable process, are easier for the retirees than abrupt departures, at least initially. Except for certain categories of single women, financial problems prove less significant than anticipated (but a niggling concern about long-term financial stability persists for many). The concluding chapter offered some advice—*that's not why I'm reading you, Dr. Weiss, nor why I'm writing my book*—which questioned the wisdom of moving far away for a better climate or to be closer to children. The problem with relocating is that although it may be easy to cultivate new acquaintances, it can be hard to make new friends with whom to have a deep and rich social life.

* * *

Two weeks later, back at my writer's group, Justin eyed me during the general check-in when we share news at the beginning of the session. "I followed a lead about a guy for you to interview for your retirement project, Bob, but I struck out. I thought he was a brilliant prospect, but, boy, was I barking up the wrong tree." Heads perked up around the table.

I took the bait. "In what way?"

"He's at least sixty-five, a fairly private person, and had a responsible job. One day, he's a full-time employee, not much else going on in his life. The next day, he's retired and everything stops. His friends worry about him. They invite him to dinner, encourage him to try some activities, and more or less try to look out for him, but he's evasive. Polite, but doesn't pick up on any of the suggestions."

I sighed. "Yeah, that's a type of person I'd like to interview. But they're not necessarily willing to talk. Not many people like telling the world that things aren't going so great in their life, and that it's probably their own fault."

Justin shook his head slowly from side to side. "No, unwillingness to talk wasn't the issue at all." He gave a lopsided grin. "Turns out, he's had a little woman, young enough to be his granddaughter, on the side for at least a couple of years. He kept her secret because he thought his family would be scandalized about her. He was right. When the secret spilled, they were aghast and shunned him."

"How did they find out?" someone asked.

"I don't know. The only other thing I know is that the couple has apparently just left town to live abroad. Probably in one of those expat communities in Mexico or Thailand where the living is cheap and the weather warm."

"Too bad for me," I said. "Sounds like he'd have a great story to tell." I paused as I realized the man would probably have been out of scope for my project. "But maybe the story belongs elsewhere. I managed to squeeze in Gillian, who said she was emotionally single, but the secretly-not-single would really be pushing the boundary."

ANDREW

When I finally found a suitable man to interview, he balked. Strongly.

"No, you shouldn't include my story," Andrew declared. "I'm too much of an oddball case."

"Well, I don't think you're all that strange," I countered. "I wouldn't have asked if I thought you odd." Andrew may have been over sixty, but his slender frame could have been that of a forty-year-old. His thinning, grey-brown hair placed him in perhaps his fifties. Divorced, but psychologically healthy as far as I could tell. Active and bright. He seemed quite normal to me.

"No, I mean my situation was peculiar, not that I'm personally strange."

"How so?"

"My original thought was that maybe I could start my retirement two or three years hence by returning to school for an advanced degree. Yes, I admit it's nerdy, but school is something I'm good at and enjoy. I floated this idea by a professor I know. She not only encouraged me, but somehow persuaded me to apply for a program whose deadline was in just ten days time. Ten days! I had to come up with people who had academic credibility to serve as references, dream up a statement about my research topic, gather transcripts, and so on. Then, to my horror, I was admitted."

Now I was really puzzled. "What? That sounds like good news to me."

"Horror," he said, "because this was the wrong time in my life. I was still working full-time. However, I didn't want to turn down the offer because there was no guarantee I'd get a second chance in a few years' time—a lot depends on the strength of the applicant pool each year. Perhaps I had benefited from exceptionally lacklustre competition this year, and I wasn't prepared to relocate to attend some other university that might accept me in the future.

"Okay, now I'm getting it. I understand your concern about competitive admissions." I took a sip of coffee, waiting for whatever Andrew would say next, but he just sat in silence. Finally, I asked what happened.

"Only at that point did I look in any detail at the program requirements. I realized I could get through the first year by taking just one daytime course per semester. I, fortunately, had a fair amount of vacation and professional development time and more flexibility in my work schedule than many people, so I managed to juggle my timetable to play at being a student one day a week. This dual life went on for eighteen months. Then I retired to become a full-time student."

He peered at me. "Do you know anybody else who comes vaguely close to having a similar experience?" A look of smug satisfaction spread across his lightly tanned face. He evidently thought he had bested me.

I ignored his question, commenting instead that his life sounded plenty full, and that perhaps *play* wasn't quite the right word for graduate studies.

"Yes, it was entirely appropriate in my case," Andrew corrected me. "I was the epitome of a slacker student, studying in the same field I had worked in for over three decades. On some topics, I knew more than the instructors. I already had lots of data that I could use in a thesis. There was no stress because, unlike in my twenties, I wasn't hoping to get a job as a result of my studies. If things didn't go well, I could simply quit, and there'd be no bad consequences. Plus, I was still working and had no financial concerns. Later, my pension covered my living and other expenses.

"All in all, it was rather agreeable, but unusual. I hadn't planned it this way. One thing led to another. Things just kept working out. I doubt anybody else would ever have a similar experience."

"Okay, maybe your situation was indeed unique," I conceded, "but I suspect parts of your story are universal. For example, you started thinking at some point about retiring. When and how did that happen?"

Andrew must have been asked this question several times before because he immediately launched into an explanation. Partly, he genuinely wanted to return to university, and partly his workplace was changing in ways that he didn't especially like. He added, "Although being in a job that had become slightly dissatisfying may have been sufficient to get me thinking about retirement, it wasn't enough to actually make me leave. I needed to know I was moving towards something, not merely stepping away from work. That's why I went to see the professor in the first place. I wanted to know if another degree was something I could transition into."

"Could you tell me more about your notion of a transition into retirement?" I asked. "I've encountered this idea before, but I'm not sure if everybody means the same when they talk about it."

This question slowed him down. "Well, I don't know," he finally said. "I didn't want to stop working all of a sudden and then do nothing, yet part-time work wasn't an option in my job." He faltered. "I guess the other piece is that I'm a huge believer in doing something new each year. Keeps you fresh and on your toes. It's a question of balance, of having some familiar, long-term activities that ground you, but also a few new things to avoid slipping into a rut. When you're retired, you don't have job duties or kids forcing you to step outside your comfort zone. So, I thought I had to be intentional about trying new things."

"And would you say you made a successful transition?"

"Oh, yes, way better than I anticipated. Being a student turned out to be a multi-year transition into retirement, with structure and responsibilities slipping away gradually."

"In what ways?"

"First, I still had to take a few courses, so that meant schedules and deadlines, but not a full-time course load. Then I had to do what are called comprehensive exams. In some departments, those are intensive oral exams, but in my program, it meant spending a semester writing three big papers on broad questions along the lines of the meaning of life and the nature of the universe. I had a deadline for these papers, but I had to come up with my own schedule and process for writing them. Finally came the thesis. I could go at whatever pace I wanted, in whatever manner I wanted. It kept me well occupied, but now everything I did was up to me, rather than somebody else telling me what to do. At least, until my supervisory committee read the draft and suggested the types of changes I should make."

I remembered that my original question had been about Andrew's decision-making regarding retirement. I still didn't feel I had a complete answer, even though I knew when he had retired. "Had you made up your mind about retirement when you started your studies, or did you decide later on?"

"I told you that I started off doing one course a term."

"Yes."

"That was fine, except that it might take me a decade to complete the program at that pace. The university said I had to finish in six or seven years. So, after a year or so in the program, I had to decide if I was serious about my studies. I decided I was, and my job satisfaction was still merely adequate. Paid employment now seemed highly overrated, whereas I enjoyed my classmates, most of whom were in their thirties and forties. So, I gave my notice at work, but it didn't feel like retirement when the time came. More like switching jobs. I went from a job where I was a worker to a job where I was a student. And then I eventually eased out of student life with a couple of tiny consulting contracts. That's how I slowly came to be where I am today, blissfully out of the labour market, as well as not in school. It happened very slowly and gently."

❋   ❋   ❋

When I first approached Andrew, I expected he would articulately describe his behaviour. I didn't know him well enough, though, to have a sense of how open he would be to sharing his regrets and vulnerabilities. Two introverted guys chatting at a patio café—not an auspicious prospect for drilling down to the emotions that really matter in a person's life. At least the weather was nice and the beverages good, a consolation if the conversation remained casual rather than deep.

"And now that all that is behind you," I asked gingerly, "how is retirement treating you? Is it what you expected or hoped it would be?"

He shrugged and smiled a little. "Really, I haven't found retirement to be a big deal, perhaps because I eased into it so gradually. I'm basically the same person living much the same type of life I've always had. I just have a whole lot more time now."

"And does time ever weigh heavily for you?" I held my breath, wondering if Andrew would admit that it sometimes did, or whether he'd shut down this line of inquiry altogether.

Although he avoided answering me, he did make a comment I thought significant. "It's easy to keep busy. Finding activities that are meaningful and life-giving, now that's a different matter. Being busy and being fulfilled are not necessarily the same thing. In a similar vein, I've done some great travelling, but that's just an interlude. It's icing on the cake, and too much icing gets sickly. It's in my day-to-day life that I find my purpose for living, not during the few weeks, once or twice a year, when I'm in an exotic place."

"This sounds important. Tell me more."

Andrew pursed his lips, then brightened up. "Take volunteering, for example. Lots of places are only too happy to have you come and relieve their staff from doing trivial, time-consuming tasks. Now, I'm the first to admit that sometimes it's nice to do mindless chores so that you can meet and chat with others, all the more if you're helping in some small way to make the world a better place while you socialize. But sometimes, it's just boring, low-level, busy-work. At the other extreme, sometimes organizations want you to commit too much time, take on too much responsibility, or be tied down to a rigid schedule. This starts to feel like work, except you're not getting paid.

"I've found it harder than I expected to discover volunteer roles in the middle. Roles that are sufficiently challenging and interesting, that bring me into contact with people I enjoy, but which aren't too burdensome."

"I see what you're getting at."

Andrew continued, "Or take recreational programs. There's dozens and dozens of things you can register for. Only a few of them, though, will be right for you, and sometimes, it takes trial and error to figure out which those might be. If you stick with only your familiar activities, you'll probably eventually become bored or dull. You have to experiment with a few new activities, and those don't always work out."

I asked what some of his experiments had been. Beginner pickleball lessons had turned out to be a big hit. He elaborated, "I had thought pickleball was an activity for out-of-shape people who would shortly be carpet bowling and playing bingo, but it's fast, fun, and a good cardio and flexibility workout." He qualified, "If you're reasonably athletic and slightly competitive, that is." This new sport was growing so rapidly in popularity, though, that getting court time was becoming a problem. Andrew wasn't willing to queue up to play, and so he had set pickleball aside, at least for the time being.

He then ordered me not to laugh at his next experiment, as he sheepishly admitted to having started Zumba dance in recent months. "The Latin hip moves are loosening my muscles in a very healthy way, even if I do look rather dorky. Fortunately, half the class is just as bad as I am, so I simply laugh as I try with varying success to imitate the fast-paced moves. I go to stay supple and for the aerobic workout, not so much because I want to dance. But I have to admit, it's fun and the hour flies by."

Andrew's demeanour is so conservative that I had to stifle my laughter; this flamboyant revelation seemed so out of character. Give him credit, though—he was practicing what he preached about broadening during retirement. "I'm sometimes the only male in the class, so I get kudos just for showing up and giving it a shot. Expectations of males in dance are so low, mostly for good reason, that I see eyebrows rising when I can keep up, even if I'm not pretty."

"Wow," I said, "you're becoming a different person in your retirement."

"Not really. This is who I've always been. It's more that people have only seen parts of me and are surprised when I reveal other aspects of who I am." He became more serious. "But there is indeed something that I'm finding a little new and strange. This is the first time when I've ever felt I could do absolutely whatever I wanted in my life."

"I'm not sure I'm catching what you mean. We always have choices."

"When you're young, for sure you have choices about education and careers, but, nonetheless, there's an expectation that you're going to do something. There's social pressure to find a partner. Then, if marriage comes along, there's a script for a house and kids. Whether you choose to follow that script is, of course, up to you, but it's a frame of reference. And, regardless of whatever you choose or are forced to do, you still have to generate enough income to live on. There may be family to care for, and so on.

"In my retirement, all that has disappeared. I can do whatever I want because I don't have any family obligations—my kids are well launched in their own lives, and all my parents' generation are dead. I don't need to generate an income. I'm not constrained by health issues. That absolute freedom feels a little weird. I'm not saying it's good or bad, just that it's a new sensation for me. I haven't felt overwhelmed by all the choice and lack of societal guidance for living this phase of life, but I can understand why some retirees freeze at first and don't know where to begin."

I used Andrew's comment about other people to shift into a discussion as to how retirement was affecting his friendships and social connections. His first observation was to say that he was ambivalent about being with seniors. "Not all old people act or think old, but some really do. I don't look my age, so perhaps it's just vanity that makes me mildly uncomfortable being part of a group that is obviously senior. But sometimes I join such groups because they're convenient and fun. I guess I'm just reluctant to admit that I'm a senior, and these are now my peers."

"What about your relationships with younger people?" I asked. "The reason I'm wanting to know about your social life is that I've heard that the married tend to do better in retirement than the unmarried. It could be that people who live alone are more vulnerable to social isolation."

Andrew thought for a moment before saying that his retired status probably affected his social life less than did his psychological makeup. "I'm quite comfortable with my own company and doing things by myself, which is clearly beneficial when one lives alone. I don't feel the need to always have a companion in order to do something. But it would be easy for me to slip into isolation, and that's not a good thing. We need other people in our lives. People who challenge and broaden us, let alone care about us. I think my independence is simultaneously a strength and a weakness. I'm having to be more intentional about meeting people now than when I was working."

He smiled when he said he hoped he wasn't about to say something sexist, but he believed males don't connect with each other as well as women do. "And my limited experience of trying simply to be friends with women is that things tend to get complicated. Too often, there's somebody in the background either hoping or fearing it's a budding romance. I wish ordinary companionship across the sexes was easier in our society."

Picking up the gender theme, I mentioned having read that men tend to do a little better in the period immediately after leaving work. "Perhaps," I opined, "it's because their workmates weren't especially supportive emotionally, so there isn't much to miss." But it's women who apparently do better in the long run, the theory being, as Andrew had suggested, that they more easily establish new friendships. "But," I cautioned, "I haven't seen anything suggesting these differences between the sexes are all that great, at least not if one sets aside the major financial problems that some single, retired women face as the result of their marriage ending."

"That makes sense," Andrew said. He eyed me intently as he changed topics, circling back to where our conversation had begun. "And does it now make sense to you, Bob, why you definitely shouldn't include my story in your project? You've managed to get an interview out of me, but the only parts that might be relevant for your readers are hardly newsworthy. Like mindless busyness not being fulfilling, and considering retirement because work was becoming less fun. The few interesting parts of my experience were unusual and don't transfer well."

"I now understand your point of view entirely," I replied. "It seems pretty reasonable. Thanks for being patient enough to explain it to me."

We carried our empty mugs to a trolley just inside the double door, said our leave-takings, and wound our separate ways through the parking lot.

CYNTHIA

I met Cynthia through our respective writing groups. She perked up as I described my first-year-of-retirement project to those present, and her reactions heartened me. "Would you consider doing an interview with me?" I eventually asked. "It's perfectly fine to say no because the conversation goes better when people are keen and not merely being nice to me. I have a little write-up about the project to help you decide if an interview appeals to you."

Cynthia agreed, and now I hoped she wouldn't turn out to be another person who had worked in health care. I knew my pool of interviewees would never be well balanced, but I wanted it to be somewhat diverse. "No, not in health," she assured me. "I retired from an administrative job in a social services department." Evidently, I have a thing for government employees because I wasn't attracting a lot of interviewees from the private and not-for-profit sectors.

Her next comment made me hesitate. "I've had a pretty ordinary life. Nothing out of the normal has happened to me. I've made some notes based on the sample questions in your handout, but I don't have much to say."

"I wouldn't be too sure about that," I replied stoically. "Let's see what emerges. My experience with these interviews is that it doesn't matter how much drama people have had in their lives, the resulting stories are always interesting because they're so very real." A thought crossed my mind. "Maybe I'm confusing you with somebody else, but didn't you once say you had an alcoholic husband?"

"Yes. It took me a long time to reach the decision, but I probably would have kicked him out if he hadn't died first."

"And that didn't have any impact on what you'll tell me during the interview?"

She reflected for a while. "No, not really. I've been pretty fortunate."

Clearly there was more to Cynthia than met the eye, perhaps even more than she herself realized. Was she incredibly well adjusted or just naïve?

*　　*　　*

Cynthia said that she had enjoyed her job and the people she worked with. The main drawback was that she despised the commute to and from work.

"But you retired voluntarily," I said. "Most people would have just whined about the commuting and kept on working. Or perhaps moved closer to work. Surely there was more to it for you?"

As Cynthia talked, I realized that retirement appealed to her not in order to escape her workplace but as a way of making time to do the things she valued. "Another consideration was that I really like to travel, and I wanted to be able to travel whenever I felt like it, rather than wait for those two or three weeks each year. Writing was also on my list of things to do. I had started, but life got in the way. Having a grandchild coming also helped."

"It's sounding like you're one of those people whose first association with the word *retirement* is freedom."

"Oh, yes. Definitely. Being able to do something if and when I want to. And if I don't feel like doing anything, sometimes I'll just sit at home most of the day and watch TV, or work on my stories, or play computer games. Just because I can. I don't feel the obligation to go out and do things."

"You're in a different headspace than some retirees. Some feel guilty or lost in their freedom or, perhaps, think that they're wasting time."

"Not me." She pulled her blue-framed glasses off her face and held them to the light, apparently trying to figure out whether it was worth cleaning the lenses. She continued. "When I had a bad cold a while ago, I took the whole week off to get well. Didn't do a thing. You can't do that when you're working because you feel obliged to go to the office, if it's at all possible."

"But wasn't that an anomaly? You're not ill all the time."

"Of course. I live at a leisurely pace most of the time, not like the total sloth I was that week." She described her delight at indulging in the Vancouver Film Festival, attending whenever she felt so inclined rather than going only after work. "Likewise, I've been able to do a couple of day trips with my grandkids, accompanying them on school outings."

Having a sense now of why she had wanted to retire, I was curious about the process of ending employment. "So, at some point, you started thinking seriously about retiring?"

"Yes. About two years before I turned sixty, I had to dream up some goals for my next performance review with my supervisor. I realized I'd had enough, so I wrote that my goal was to retire in two years." Her superiors clucked about this because she had a lot of corporate knowledge that they didn't want to lose. They cajoled and encouraged her to stay longer. "I just stuck to my guns."

"How did you feel during that last stretch at work?"

"It was mainly a matter of documenting what I was carrying around in my head. I made a binder of things, notes and examples. I've been back to visit several times, and for the first year, I'd say that my desk remained the same. It was quite funny."

"So, it was low drama at the end?"

"Oh, yes. That's the way my life has been most of the time." As an afterthought, she described a touch of sadness during her last week. "Mostly because I liked my coworkers and would miss seeing them each day." It wasn't only the people, though, that she mourned. A new process promised to change her job significantly. "I was sorry I wouldn't be there to see how it worked out."

If I had aspirations of turning Cynthia's retirement story into a potboiler, it didn't seem that she was going to help in any way. She just reiterated that she had reached the point where she was ready to do what she wanted, when she wanted, so she called it quits at work. If I desired tension in this tale, I concluded that I'd have to look for it elsewhere. "Maybe we should turn now to your first year of retirement."

"Let's see, I retired in January. In February, I took a

cruise with friends—I've never cruised on my own—to Australia and New Zealand. In November, I moved, and you know how much work packing entails. So, things happened that year, but at a comfortable pace, according to my own schedule. I didn't just stop and do nothing.

"I guess that downsizing was my big event in that first year. I yearned for a rancher after having lived in a two-storey. It was either Richmond or out this way, and I didn't want to live in Richmond. My daughter lived in Surrey, and I ended up close by her, in Langley.

"The only thing that went wrong, and it wasn't a major thing, was that when I put my house up for sale, it didn't sell." *Not a major thing to be saddled with an extra home,* I thought incredulously, but I bit my tongue so that Cynthia could continue. "I got a renter in for a while. The house didn't sell until August of the following year, for a little less than I wanted. But the price was still above what I had paid, so I was ahead in the game. It was just a bit frustrating that it took so long. But that's life. Things happen and you deal with them. The delay and price didn't throw me off."

Cynthia sat placidly, waiting for my next question, while I made a mental note to return to her low-key philosophy later in the interview. I suspected some gems remained to be unearthed.

"Did moving prove to be a good decision? I gather that retirees have mixed results with this."

"Oh, yes. I like it." She talked about the pleasure of being close to her grandkids, but that she had made it clear that she wouldn't become a permanent babysitter. "Just an emergency contact. I know some people who are regular babysitters, and their lives are very restricted. I love to travel with my friends. This way I can get up and go whenever I want."

There's the freedom theme again.

I asked if she had plugged into the local community right away.

"It was hard at first," she conceded, "because I didn't know anybody. I joined the seniors' centre to meet people and have been going there for six years. I met my neighbours. My neighbours have changed, but I've kept in touch with the original ones, and the new ones are great. I volunteered with the RCMP doing Speed Watch because a friend did it in her area, and she found it interesting. My role in it has changed over time, but it has become part of my routine."

She said she'd think about my community connections question for a moment but said nothing more. Eventually, she smiled, cocked her head, and reiterated, "You see, I have an ordinary, normal life. Nothing exciting happens. The most excitement I've had in the last little while is that I saw a bear at Hallowe'en."

I said I was glad that she wasn't apologizing for being ordinary. Lots of people crave a normal life. "And it sounds like you not only have family close by, but you have good relations with them. That's totally ordinary and totally wonderful."

Cynthia picked up on the topic of her daughters. "They were nine and thirteen when their dad died. The younger one moved out the year I retired. But after I bought my rancher, each of them and their husbands lived with me for one to three months, at different times, while they waited to get into their own new homes. The worst thing that happened, while one family was with me, took place when they parked their car outside during the winter. The rats got into the wiring and chewed on it, causing some problems. The other family did all the cooking, which was nice—I missed that when they moved out. So, yes, I'm blessed that we do okay as a family."

We sat in comfortable silence. Cynthia ended up being the one to break it. "You asked in your handout what the good things were in retirement. Pretty much everything. The bad? I don't really have anything bad. Like I said, I'm a very boring person when it comes to life experiences. Not too many surprises, and I don't think I'd do anything differently. That's all I have to say. Do you have more questions?"

❋　❋　❋

As a matter of fact, I did have more questions. Tons of them. But they weren't about retirement itself. Rather, they concerned the outlook that enabled Cynthia to navigate retirement so successfully.

Where to start? One's philosophy of life is not easy to articulate, and I had no idea what sorts of questions would work best. I defaulted to the tried and true, crassly asking, instead, whether money had been much of a factor in Cynthia's planning and retirement experiences.

"Yes, in a good way," she began. "The key to my early retirement was that I could afford to leave. I'm so thankful for some inheritances that have allowed me to do so much. Several relatives died, which was good for me financially, but I do miss the people. And I'm fortunate to have several small pensions, including the old age security that everybody gets.

"I've been lucky financially. My husband made enough money that I could be a stay-at-home mom, albeit generally feeling like a single parent. Even after he died, I got by on part-time work and didn't go full-time until later. Today, most new moms are back at work within the year."

Gratitude, I thought! That's one of the keys to understanding what makes Cynthia tick. How could I tease out more on this topic?

I noted that lone parents sometimes struggle financially when they reach their senior years. "I'm glad that hasn't been your situation."

"Yes," Cynthia agreed. "I have a friend older than me who still has to work because of a bad divorce, yet she has heart problems and is awaiting surgery. Why her and not me? I wonder about this, but I don't worry about it. I'm just aware that I have no reason to be unhappy.

"I've said it several times already, but I count myself very lucky that my life is so normal. I know many people who have it much worse than me. I think, how is it that their life is so difficult, and mine isn't?"

"Maybe you've done better than some people," I gently challenged, "but not everything has been wine and roses for you. You've told me that your marriage wasn't so hot, and that wasn't just a single rough patch."

Cynthia winced slightly. "Because my husband was alcoholic, I do admit there was a period when I had problems. But, in general, I kind of worked around him. And then he died, which was sad for him but not so much for me. My marriage was the worst thing that happened in my life."

"You're making something important sound trivial when you say you just worked around him. That's a big deal. Not many people can do that. Tell me more about how you managed to cope."

I'm not sure if it's possible to rattle Cynthia, but her body language suggested I had at least ruffled her a little. I hoped this would elicit something insightful.

"I started as an enabler," she murmured. "The short version is that I decided not to do that anymore." She said that she reached the point where she didn't make a fuss whether he was involved with his family or not. "I lived my life around him and, in the grand scheme of things, I was able to deal with the situation.

"I used to not talk about his alcoholism because I was ashamed. I came to the point where I just accepted it and no longer tried to hide it."

I sighed. "Shame. It's only in the last few years that I've come to understand how very damaging and debilitating it is. You deserve full credit for rising above it. I have a friend who regularly says that boldly naming problems defeats shame's power."

"Maybe," she said. "I just know that the worst part of my life ended when he passed away. I know people who have had a life a lot worse than me and are still dealing with it."

I looked Cynthia squarely in the eye. "I'm really struck that when bad things happen to you, you don't spend a lot of time pulling out your hair and asking, 'Why me?' You just seem to do whatever you have to, and move on. That's special, you know."

"Well, what's the point of doing otherwise?"

I had to admit that she was right, but it's easier to espouse her approach than to practice it. "How do you pull it off?"

"I'm not really sure why I'm like that," she responded.

Then she paused, and her eyes widened a little. I tilted my head. "I'm realizing that's not quite true. I wasn't always this way. Maybe I learned it from watching my husband. He worried about everything, ninety-nine percent of which never happened." She looked pleased with this observation. "In any event, I concluded that worrying is a waste of time and energy. Deal with things when they happen, and try not to always look for worst-case scenarios."

She nodded a little and slowly said that changing her way of thinking had served her well. I agreed. As an after-thought, she mentioned that she hadn't changed her lifestyle until years after her shift in outlook. "It's only in retirement that I've improved the way I eat. I exercise more than I used to, hoping to keep myself healthy longer."

"It sounds like you have a balanced life right now," I said. "Healthy food, exercise, some volunteering, some creative stuff, time at home…"

"Lots of travel with friends," she interjected. "I usually go on a trip each year, though one year I did three."

Time was passing, and I began looking for some con-cluding thoughts. "Do you think your years of being a stay-at-home mom helped your adjustment to retirement go so smoothly?"

"Hmmm, I don't know. I never thought about it that way." She peered at me quizzically. "I mean, I did have a job, just that it was at home."

"What I'm suggesting is that, although you needed to do things in your home and with your kids, you were in many ways self-directed. You didn't have a supervisor, or a spouse, telling you what to do next or ensuring you did things a certain way. I'm thinking that perhaps you got used to being in charge of your life, albeit within what might have been narrow confines."

"Oh, yes, that's very true." She made a few small comments about the relationship between her experiences as a mother and as a retiree, but then she took the conversation in a different direction. "As a parent, you're always second-guessing yourself about whether you've done things right or wrong in raising kids."

Even as we were winding up and saying our good-byes, I began formulating themes for my write-up. *She values freedom,* I thought, *but balances freedom with structure and routines. Careful not to get tied down by her routines. Enough money is necessary for a good retirement, but finances alone not sufficient. Also need the right attitude. It's her outlook that's key. Gratitude, and anticipating life will be good until proven otherwise. Not a status seeker.*

These are principles that all of us, retired or otherwise, would do well to adopt.

GREG

Greg's retirement is going well. "Perhaps it has to do with expectations," he mused. "If they're not met, then it's a downer." He shifted in his chair. "Maybe my expectations weren't all that high."

Greg had been a lifer, spending his entire career in the same department of an enormous organization. "We had offices in several cities, and we sometimes moved within a city when our lease came up, so it's not as if I stayed put the whole time. But my paycheque always came from the same source." He recognizes this as unusual now, but not so much in his day.

I asked when and why he had started thinking seriously about retirement. He explained about the magic number for his pension plan, a combination of age and years of service, which became the threshold for receiving a full pension. "I had thought a bit about retiring even before approaching that number, especially after attending a retirement seminar. You know, the usual stuff, like 'Am I going to be able to survive financially?' In the end, I decided simply to retire on my thirty-fifth anniversary. So, I knew my retirement date a few years in advance."

"You mean that beneath that gruff exterior, you're really a romantic at heart? You chose your quitting date mainly because you liked the poetic aptness of having exited on your thirty-fifth?"

Greg shot a glance at me and snorted. "Let's just say that I left on my own terms." He drummed his fingers twice and then locked his eyes on me.

I felt I was still on track, but that another wisecrack could side-swipe the conversation. I posed a couple of straightforward questions instead. "Did you think you'd miss the work or friendships? Were you concerned about anything as your last working day approached?"

Greg wobbled his head. "My job was okay. I liked it," he said, shrugging a little. "I didn't think I'd miss the job itself all that much. It's more that I wondered whether I might miss the people because I had some pretty good working relationships."

"And was that a big concern?"

"Not really. In contrast to a number of people I knew, I didn't think my life was defined by my job. At least, not very defined. So, I didn't worry about making the cut."

It seemed that Greg hadn't been at all anxious as retirement approached, nor did he foresee his life changing dramatically. Even though he loved to travel and continued to cruise after he retired, he has been happy to maintain his Vancouver base.

"I gave some thought to going south for the winter," he elaborated. "Perhaps spending three months in Palm Springs or Arizona. That was little more than a passing fancy. The reality is that it's not so easy to fit into those locations for an extended period when you're single."

"Which, I suppose, would also have been the case while you were working, if you had been able to take, say, a four-week winter vacation?"

"For me, yes. My friends and activities are here, and I value them."

"I'm guessing that you had a good social network, and that it just carried on when you retired."

"I would say so, yes."

While I waited to hear if he'd say more about his friendships during retirement, I noted that one side of his moustache was much greyer than the other. I started thinking about dye for facial hair and then realized I was daydreaming. Mainly to bring myself back into the conversation, I asked, "What about getting together with former colleagues during that first year?"

Greg tilted his head back and smiled. "You mean to swap war stories and refight battles?"

"Something like that."

"Yeah, I did some, but it diminished over time. Which is natural. I was invited to retirement parties and Christmas parties. Those sorts of special occasions. And I'd sometimes have lunch with individuals. It was all rather subdued, and it faded away in a healthy manner."

"Was your actual retirement day equally mellow, or did you get a lump in your throat?"

Greg described the previous weeks of clearing out his desk and delegating work. "Then there was a little party at the end, very comfortable. Nothing traumatic happened those last few days and hours."

"And then you were a retiree," I prompted.

Greg sat quietly, waiting for a question to follow this statement. When none came, he volunteered, "People have asked me if it took long to adjust to retirement. My flippant answer is, 'Yeah, maybe fifteen minutes.'"

※　※　※

Greg had thrived in his occupation, taking his workload in stride and not investing emotionally in the dramas of corporate life. He hadn't felt the need to start retirement by resting, nor did he rush to occupy all his newly available hours. Nonetheless, his time filled up. At a leisurely pace, that is.

"Fairly soon, I was doing a few things I hadn't been able to do so easily when I was working," he said. "Some were altogether new. For example, I took on a little volunteer role about a month after retiring, and I'm still doing it. It's just some bookkeeping and making a bank deposit for a non-profit. We do it in teams of two for one full morning. That's not a huge time commitment, but it was something new and forces me to get up early at least one day each week—early for me, that is, because I'm not an early riser. It keeps me in touch with other volunteers and the office staff. I enjoy both the people and the task."

"I'm curious what other new directions you ventured into."

Greg looked vacant for a moment and then mentioned that a former boss, who had retired a few months ahead of him, recalled Greg's interest in French. The boss had found some part-time work at a company that needed documents translated. He steered a few months' work to Greg. "It wasn't a game changer. But it was something I wouldn't have been able to do before. The work dried up once I finished the documents."

He said that quite a few former colleagues did return to work after retiring. "On a contractual basis or something. I didn't want to do that." He threw up his hands. "I'd had thirty-five years of doing it. No, I didn't bite when they wiggled the hook in front of me a couple of months after I left."

Greg shifted topics by saying he had rummaged out his old calendar before coming to talk with me. "Gee, I was really busy. As soon as I left work, there were new things to do. Thought I'd take some courses. Didn't happen." One of his first social engagements had been to host a cousin and his wife when his niece got married. "People came out from the east and stayed a number of days after the reception."

By now, I was seeing the general contours of Greg's first year of retirement. There had been a few little trips, then a major one that required considerable planning, a new volunteer role, the translation job, and the wedding. Now I sought specifics about an ordinary week, about the ways in which he typically spent his time.

"I go out every day. On occasion, it might only be to the store because I don't keep much food on hand and have to shop daily. I know which stores are best for which products. I do the rounds, not one big shop at a single grocery store."

Greg lives downtown and eventually sold his car after he retired. "It's been several years since I've driven even a rental car. Needless to say, I haven't joined one of the car co-ops that are so big in Vancouver." He remarked that coming out to the suburbs on transit to see me now counted as a mini-excursion in his world.

I noted that he seemed to have some structure in his life. "Not a lot, but enough to ground you. Your volunteer and church activities." My voice trailed off.

Greg picked up the ball. "Yes. I have some social engagements that carried over from when I was working. On Friday evenings, I always have something. Saturday afternoons. Keeps you thinking ahead and planning. These help."

✹ ✹ ✹

Twelve months of retirement slipped by with Greg barely noticing them. "I was sort of surprised," he said, "that time seemed to go even faster than when I was employed. Even chores like housework that I'd squeeze in when I was working, all of a sudden, I didn't have to cram them in. As a result, they quite often didn't get done. With no urgency from a tight schedule, I kept putting them off, thinking I'd do them when I felt like it."

Whereas some of his peers have told him they're a little under-stimulated, Greg hasn't found boredom to be an issue. "At most, it's a slight paralysis in deciding what to do next. I could do this, or that, or that. These things either need to be done or I want to do them, but I seem to take my time in deciding what's the most important to me at any given moment." Perhaps this is where his expectations, or lack of expectations, about the shape of his day or week affect whether he's satisfied at any particular instance. And, yes, Greg is a laidback guy, the type who would people-watch in a long queue rather than fret about the delay. So, personality must be another component of the boredom equation.

"The days go by so fast," Greg reiterated. "Sometimes

I wonder at the end of the day, 'What have I done?' It's not that I'm sitting around watching television. I guess this isn't a bad thing." One of his subtle glints surfaced and the corners of his mouth twitched. "Well, I'm not sure whether it's a bad thing or good thing." He then spoke more seriously. "I'm actually not clear whether I'm taking longer to do things than when I was working, or whether I just have the sense that I take longer."

"In any event, it doesn't sound like your life is stressful," I said.

"No."

"Was there anything you could have done without during that first year?"

Greg remained silent for an uncomfortably long period. "I don't remember anything negative, or feelings of regret, or that maybe I should have stayed a little longer. I never felt that way," he finally answered.

I believed him, so I moved on to a fresh topic. "Did you sense that people were viewing you differently?"

This, too, led to a lull in the conversation. "Yes, I guess."

"In what ways?"

"I'm having a hard time with this question. Here's a general comment about retirement, one that applies to more than just the first year." He tented his fingers and raised them to his chin. "Sometimes, it's like you have to justify your existence. I get asked 'What do you do?' It's almost an impertinent question, but it's a common one."

I nodded, thinking back to Bronwyn's comment about getting annoyed when asked how she spent her time, even when she knew the intent of the question was genuine and not accusatory.

"Maybe I'm overly sensitive about this," Greg continued, "because I sometimes wonder whether I should be doing more than I am. But I do spend a fair amount of time on volunteer work, and this has grown over time. My church involvement has also grown, and I'm finding it increasingly meaningful. I'm content. So, I figure if I have enough activities to keep me engaged and I'm happy, why rock the boat? But then that same niggling question about doing more comes back, and I repeat the cycle."

He sat more upright, widening his eyes. "I don't want you to think I'm neurotic. This isn't a big deal. It's just a little thing I sometimes wonder about."

"Relax," I assured him. "I get it. We all have things we keep circling back to."

"Yeah. Apparently, everybody's somewhere on the OCD spectrum."

"In a nutshell," I summarized, "you had a pretty smooth first year and subsequently as well?"

"Yes." He leaned forward and dropped his head. "Boring, right? Let's face it, I don't even have a smartphone to keep me in the fast lane."

I agreed immediately. "You betcha. I'm going to have to invent some inner turmoil for your write-up. That's why what I'm doing is called creative nonfiction." I couldn't quite interpret Greg's reaction, but I guessed that he was taking my tongue-in-cheek comment the way I intended. "Actually, it's really nice to hear that things are going well for you. I'm sure I'll have some readers who need reassuring that life can go on without a big disruption after employment ends."

The interview completed, we moved on to other topics.

We almost returned to retirement when we discussed people we knew who seem to have lost the skill of going out and trying new things, but somehow we ended up talking instead about new transit routes and the Canadian Longitudinal Study on Aging. After half an hour, Greg slipped on his shoes, remembered his umbrella, and made his way to the elevator.

SHELLEY

My interviewing finished, and a conclusion coming along nicely, when what to my wondering eyes should appear but the skeleton of another half chapter. Half, because this unexpected gift arrived as a monologue rather than a dialogue, just one side of a hypothetical conversation. Fortunately, it was the portion that mattered.

It also came in written form rather than orally, and it spanned four years of retirement rather than only the first year, but I wasn't going to be persnickety about these unfortunate details. The important thing was that the author, to the best of my recollection, had been single when she retired. I was confident I could make use of Shelley's information, toning down those pesky problems to better match the contours of my project. I'd start by inserting my commentary into her story, in the hope of creating the illusion of something resembling a conversation.

Shelley had been a columnist at a large-circulation newspaper, the *Vancouver Sun*. I was one of the faithful and often skimmed her columns. The topics sometimes concerned everyday activities, her own life in particular. I recalled that she loved her grandkids and lived in a heritage house—or, at least, a character house—just a few blocks from where I worked for many years. I wouldn't say I knew her writing well, but she resembled a long-time neighbour with whom you chat each time you meet at the mailbox.

Four years ago, she retired at age sixty-three. "When, after forty-one years in the newspaper business, a generous buyout offer came up, I took the money and ran. Loved my job, but I was done."

Now, she had resurfaced. The headline on March 24, 2020, proclaimed, "The Art of Idleness," and the subheading elaborated, "In her debut Life in the 60s column, Shelley Fralic touts a slower pace."

I liked the article, but it seemed a touch disingenuous. She had claimed, "And so, four years on, the art of my idleness is near fully perfected." One might think she had entirely tuned out and dropped out, especially after she depicted her bliss at waking to face another weightless day, but she hadn't. Any writer who can suddenly reappear to thousands of readers hasn't completely relinquished her former professional identity, nor has she been one hundred percent idle.

Nonetheless, she made a persuasive case for slowing down, and she captured well the yearnings of so many people when they contemplate life after work. Her point of view and her experiences deserved a place in this compendium.

✳   ✳   ✳

"You're retiring?" the article began. "Why? Won't you be bored?" Shelley said these questions "usually uttered in one breathless sentence, along with a look of confused disbelief, are delivered in a high-pitched, incredulous tone."

Why, I've heard others ask in a similar vein, would somebody leave while at the top of their game, or when they still had so much to contribute? Sometimes accusatory, sometimes solicitous, the implication is that one is giving up on life.

I could picture her amusement with what she described as shock and awe in her circle. "What was I thinking? Giving up a great career, good money, pensionable years, extended benefits. Surely I was mad."

Then came the article's pivotal question and answer. "And, good Lord, what would I do with myself all day long? The answer to that last question was easy: Nothing."

Nothing. We've heard from others in this book that not everybody finds it easy to do little or nothing, even when they believe that's what they desire. And while none of my interviewees currently complained of boredom, the research indicates that tedium and disorientation are common enough in retirement, at least for a stretch. So, doing nothing is neither risk free nor as simple as it seems.

It turned out that Shelley isn't doing absolutely nothing, either. It might be more accurate to say she is doing very different things, in a very laid-back manner. "Oh, there is the morning routine of coffee and newspapers at the local café. The visits with mom, who is ninety-three and still doing daily floor exercises. There are pies to bake, documentaries to watch, beaches to stroll, books to finish, family to spoil, sales to shop." That sounds to me like a relaxed and engaged person who has found meaning at the neighbourhood level, one whom I envy a little.

The external pressure to remain hyperactive in retirement, a pressure some of my interviewees had internalized, is substantial. "Make no mistake," Shelley wrote, "one must have a purpose. There shall be no wasting of the day, no lollygagging in the remaining years." As a result, some retirees travel relentlessly, punishing their bodies and finances, "haunted by that silly bucket list. We journey to Machu Picchu and Iceland and Slovenia, coasting waterways on kitted-out barges, riding tough terrain on flimsy bicycles, and wearing unflattering fast-wicking Lycra and goofy toques."

The sources of that pressure are undoubtedly multiple, but Shelley chose to draw her readers' attention to just one, the guilt baby boomers feel for having led such privileged lives. They are, in her words, the golden generation. "The covenant? Thou must not squander one single second of our good fortune."

Nuts to this, Shelley argued. I'm not sure whether it's hyperbole or whether she truly believes it, but she called for her fellow retirees to do nothing, gladly and boldly embracing idleness. "And really, wasn't that the point of retiring? You work for fifty years, get the kids through piano lessons and acne, transfer your caretaking obligations to elderly parents and—if you are especially blessed—continue to nurture the astonishing love you have for your grandchildren."

Towards the end of the column, Shelley briefly mentioned another theme, one about choice and self-determination, which I hoped she'd explore in a future piece. When your body slows, she said, and what once mattered to you and to others, "really doesn't matter anymore, you realize that it's time to do what you want to do, not what is expected of you."

Now, that's a retirement mantra worth repeating. "It's time to do what you want to do, not what is expected of you." Yes, self-absorption poses a slight danger, and it has a way of decaying you from within. The benefits, though, of living authentically, especially if you harbour even a mild awareness and fondness for others, can be significant.

For many retirees, their authentic self notices the roses and makes a point of smelling them. It is less concerned with what others might think, choosing instead to nurture the inner child. It perhaps sees the glass as half-full more often than half-empty. And it saunters along at a comfortable pace.

FINAL THOUGHTS

Despite the snippets of conversation and readings that reverberated endlessly in my mind, I never did detect any themes unique to single retirees. The stories singles told me about beginning their new phase of life also seemed pertinent to married people. I eventually decided that factors other than marital status, such as expectations and lifestyle choices, must be much more telling influences on one's contentment in the first year of retirement.

Had I therefore defined the scope of this little book too narrowly by focusing on singles? I think not. By highlighting the stories of single people, the spotlight stayed on the effects of starting retirement, uncomplicated by all the relationship issues in a marriage. So, although the book's scope was okay, my audience was clearly broader than I had envisaged. I had written *about* singles, but it turned out to be *for* everybody.

Now I became curious about whether the reverse might be true. If the retirement experiences of singles can help married retirees navigate better, what might singles learn from the married? My musings eventually led me to look up *retired husband syndrome*, a cute term I had encountered several times in the previous months. As I learned about the syndrome's symptoms, though, I came to see them as ominous rather than endearing.

Early in the 1990s, medical and sociological researchers began describing stress-related physical illnesses and depression that afflicted over half of Japan's older female population. Skin rashes, asthma, ulcers, and high blood pressure developed at abnormally high rates in these women. The emergence of their physical and psychological symptoms correlated with the retirement of their husbands—men who had typically worked long hours and socialized primarily with their colleagues. All of a sudden, a woman could find herself housebound with a demanding and bored husband, with whom she might have maintained only a superficial relationship for decades. Their cultural conditioning encouraged wives to defer to the whims of their spouses, no matter how little joy this might bring them or affect the marriage.

Japan's workaholic workplaces and traditional gender roles may have made it the epicentre for retired husband syndrome, but other countries are hardly immune from what here might better be termed *retired spouse syndrome*. According to Google, common Internet search terms in North America that are related to retired husband syndrome include "retired husband micromanages," "retired husband lazy," "bored retirement husband," "my husband is home all the time," and "retired husband has no hobbies." It seems that marriage highlights the consequences of coping poorly with retirement's predictable challenges.

One gets the impression from this line of Internet

searching that our society is suffering from an epidemic of meddling, ever-present, dependent, angry, or depressed retirees who listen poorly to their partners. Fortunately, that's an overstatement. To the extent the disease does exist, it's highly treatable with the standard relationship prescriptions that start with open, honest communication and which progress through such topics as boundaries and interdependence, self-discipline, and initiative.

The main lesson I took from my research about married retirees is that if you use work as an excuse to avoid living in a healthy and emotionally balanced manner, not taking the time or making the effort to care for your psychological well-being, then you may be setting yourself up for a nasty stint when employment disappears. Retirement doesn't cause the dysfunction in one's life or relationships so much as expose it. The abundant hours of unstructured free time provide a medium in which seeds of maladjustment can grow and flourish.

Unhappy single people can hide and live a life of quiet desperation. When, however, you're in a relationship, your partner is affected by your mood. Yes, your spouse might constructively help you get through a rocky adjustment period as you begin retirement, but they might also finally confront you about long-standing issues, now that the problems can no longer be swept under the workplace rug. So, there's plenty to ponder here.

* * *

Evidently, I was pondering way too much because, several weeks later, I still hadn't stopped contemplating how couples might illuminate the retirement paths of singles. The Internet is a sore temptation when one has an itch for knowledge, and I finally succumbed to it, yet again. Unclear as to what exactly I was looking for, I experimented with a variety of search terms. Eventually, some promising leads emerged.

The first websites I landed upon tended to discuss what must surely be the number one topic for marriage counsellors: communication. Consider anything about couples' relationship problems and, sooner or later, some sort of communication issue seems to surface. More frequent talks! Better listening! Greater authenticity! Less judgement! And so on. You know the drill, and it's all true.

Regarding retirement, the communication guidance seemed mainly to be about sharing expectations. "Instead of focusing on your retirement *from* work," said one website, "talk to each other about what you want to retire *to*." Although singles don't face the ordeal of negotiating with a partner attached to a dissimilar postretirement vision, this counsel reinforces the importance of preretirement planning by everyone. What do you want to retire *to*? If only we all had a clear answer to that question. And one that endures the reality check of the first twelve months post–employment.

Other communication advice for those in committed relationships was to take into account the needs and interests of your partner. Upon retirement, one blogger scolded, "You are now forced to do something you should have done from the day you were married: create a lifestyle that takes each other's feelings into account." In skimming the paragraphs, I saw how acknowledging one another's emotions and interests could be equally helpful for singles seeking to strengthen their friendships. In fact, anything that encourages mutual respect and sensitivity can't be bad.

I smiled about the recommendation to give one's partner a little less unsolicited advice. This transfers very well to the realm of friendship, especially to those friendships where you feel safe to divulge what's really on your mind.

A passing reference in an otherwise dull study intrigued me. The author speculated whether his data might indicate that "retirement transitions undermine married retirees' satisfaction if they enhance the other partner's influence in the relationship." I interpreted this conjecture to mean, "You're less likely to be happy if you feel you're losing power and control." This insight goes a long way towards explaining the bumps at the start of some retirements. Whether married or single, leaving one's job can mean losing the position where you had the most status and influence, where subordinates and clients listened carefully to what you said, regardless of whether they subsequently complied with your requests (which they often did).

An antidote to such diminishment is to take charge of your life, rather than playing the role of a retirement victim. We've heard this recommendation before: make retirement a time for personal growth, regardless of your marital situation. Live boldly, fail boldly, and learn to fly to new destinations. Find fresh venues in which to make a difference.

I ended my ramble through cyberspace on a haunting note when I stumbled upon a fear that I suspect is quite common, but rarely voiced. It happened to be mentioned on a marriage website, but it persists among seniors independently of marital status: the fear of dementia. My interviewees were well aware of the fragility of their physical well-being, and concern about depression lurked in the background of much that I wrote, but this was the first explicit mention of dementia that I had encountered.

The response to this anxiety was that "a healthy diet, social contact, and mental stimulation can maintain or even improve brain health. Physical health also has a huge impact on mental health." Well, hello. This sounds a lot like the other advice we've heard for a successful retirement, essentially to maintain a healthy lifestyle. Actually, it's advice for everyone.

❋   ❋   ❋

At this point, I had reached a place, if not of closure, then of having attained a decent overview of the retirement landscape. I'm still learning and finding new rabbit trails to explore, but with diminishing returns. Echoes of past conversations increasingly intermingle with my latest findings. My initial curiosity, bred in my yoga class so many months ago, has been satisfied. It's time to call it quits on this project.

So, what might I say when people, especially hesitant individuals on the verge of retirement, ask what I've discovered?

"Yes," I think I'll reply, "retirement is complex and sometimes ambiguous, but, by and large, people like being retired. It can take a few months or even years to adjust, but eventually people find their rhythm, especially if they have thought in advance about their postretirement priorities and options."

Retirees who persist in forging new friendships, who risk looking silly as they explore new activities, and who seek ways to keep contributing—people who, in short, are open, curious, and caring—tend to make their retirement a rich and rewarding stage of life. It doesn't happen automatically, but the six people I interviewed have demonstrated that a bit of common sense, patience, and effort can make launching into retirement, whether solo or together, a rewarding voyage.

CPSIA information can be obtained
at www.ICGtesting.com
Printed in the USA
BVHW032208270920
589749BV00001B/19

9 781525 585715